1% Fitness

Move Better. Train Smarter. Live Longer

Mike Sheridan

1% Fitness/Mike Sheridan
ISBN: 978-0993745591
contact@leanlivinginc.com

Contents

This book is dedicated to those that still believe they don't have time to exercise. Give me 1% of your week, and I'll give you the body you've always wanted.

"The greater your muscle mass, the lower your risk of death...rather than worrying about weight...we should be trying to maximize and maintain muscle mass."

— Dr. Arun Karlamangla

Muscle & Health

If I asked you why you don't look and feel the way you want, you'd probably answer:

"I don't have the time."

or

"I don't have the discipline."

I know this because conventional wisdom continues to give you a distorted image of what it takes to maintain an attractive physique. Like most North Americans, you've been led to believe that a better body is only achieved by eating like a bird and exercising like a maniac.

> The common approach to getting fit is leaving 75% of the population Fat and Frustrated, and the other 25% Overworked and Underfed.

The reason you continue to fall short, or burn-out in an effort to keep up, is because 'more exercise' and 'less eating' is not the solution. As I outline in *Eat Meat And Stop Jogging*, our body adjusts to a chronic energy-shortage, by increasing hunger to access more calories, stockpiling fat as a fuel reserve, and slowing our resting metabolic (energy burning) rate.

Essentially, our body learns to function on less calories per day by using less energy, and storing more. Leading to weight regain shortly after the 3, 6, or 12 week restriction period, and leaving us with damaged hormones and a disrupted metabolism for up to a year afterwards! Meaning, despite efforts to eat less and exercise more in the future, we continue to fatten.

If you haven't already, please check out Eat Meat And Stop Jogging before reading further. This is the prerequisite to 1% Fitness, because it's essential that you fully understand the nutrition and fitness misconceptions keeping North American fat and sick.

Conventional Wisdom = Under-Eat & Over-Exercise

For the last 50 years, we've been taught that improving our physique and maintaining our health requires:

- Restricting calories to lose weight
- Limiting animal protein to prevent degenerative disease
- Performing endurance exercise to burn calories

Meanwhile, all this caloric deficit and over-exercise plan does is elevate fat storage, accelerate muscle and bone loss, increase cortisol and oxidative stress, and lower immune function and reproductive health. Which, as discussed in *Eat Meat And Stop Jogging*, are all factors related to aging that we should be trying to avoid not promote.

Although many will achieve their goal of 'weight-loss' by exercising more or eating less, research suggests that nearly 40% of that weight is muscle when lost via caloric reduction. Meaning 40% less of the tissue that raises our resting metabolic (energy burning) rate, and controls nearly 60-75% of our total energy expenditure.

> A caloric-deficit (through diet or exercise) is a double-edged sword - as you continue to decrease the rate at which you burn calories, you lose useful muscle that would otherwise burn additional calories.

The less muscle you have, the less energy you burn, and the easier it is to gain. No matter how much you exercise, or how little you eat. The end result, is a high-fat low muscle physique, that's hardly aligned with why you started exercising and eating right in the first place.

One could argue that exercising to 'Burn Calories' is an even more damaging approach to getting fit as trying to eat less. Especially when that exercise choice is steady-state endurance training (cardio); which continues to be the universal choice. Largely, because we've developed the false belief that exercise should focus on burning calories, but also because we've been convinced that endurance training is best way to stay healthy and fit.

In reality, the only thing cardio promotes is the ability to run for a really long time. And aside from creating a physique that's far from ideal, this is an inferior biomarker for health and longevity.

1. Muscle Mass
2. Strength
3. Metabolic Rate
4. Body Fat Percentage
5. Aerobic Capacity

What's worse, is that cardio reduces the more critical biomarkers in the process. As those that continue to run, swim, and cycle further and more frequently in an effort to get and stay fit are losing muscle. And as it continues to decline, they're losing strength, storing fat, and decreasing their resting metabolic rate.

Lower Muscle = Lower Health Span

With no plan to prevent it, we lose 40% of our muscle mass between the ages of 50 and 80.

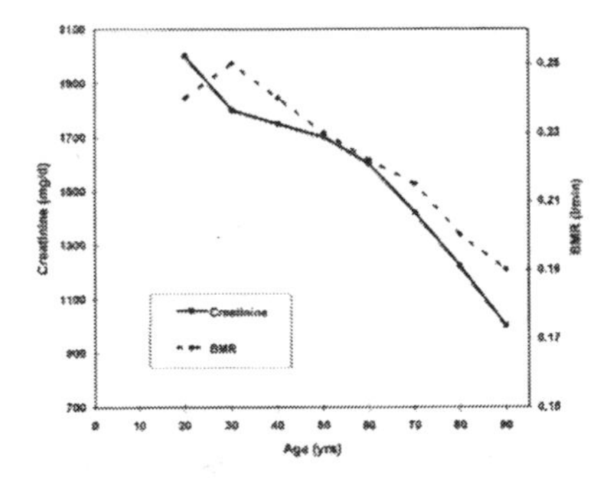

Aside from declines in physical functioning and elevations in disability and mortality, this loss of lean muscle mass (sarcopenia)

is a significant contributor to metabolic dysfunction. And regardless of body mass index, low muscle strength is predictive of mortality across all age groups over 50 (including the oldest of old – 89+).

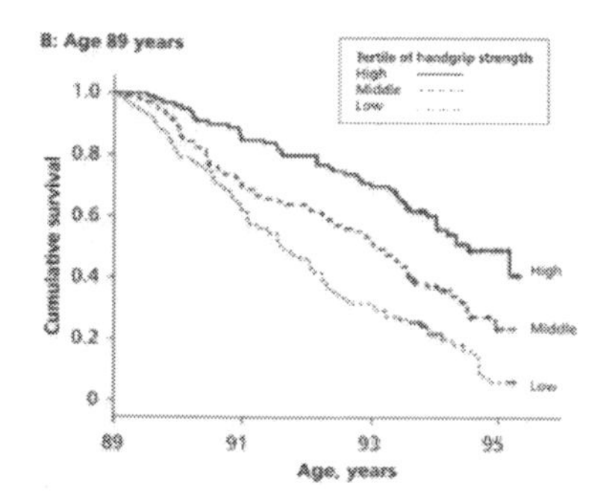

These reductions in insulin sensitivity, resting metabolic rate, and muscle protein synthesis, lead to elevated blood sugar, excess fat storage, and insulin resistance. Over time, this becomes diabetes, heart disease, cognitive impairment, and even cancer.

Basically, muscle loss and/or a lack of focus on preservation, is accelerating the aging process, and the unfortunate ailments that come with it. Whether from a physical strength and stability standpoint, or from a fat storage and metabolic disorder perspective.

Yet somehow we continue to prioritize exercise and follow diets that burn muscle? To please a scale that tells us nothing about our strength or muscle to fat percentage?

When we try to lose weight by depriving ourselves of essential nutrients, or chronically exercising to reach a deficit, we shorten our 'health span.'

> "...your lifespan—how many years you live—is important, but perhaps not as much so as your health span: that period of your life when you're functional and able to perform everyday life tasks for yourself." - Tufts University

Even though we're living longer now than ever (lifespan), research is suggesting that the majority of that extra time is spent confined to a hospital bed, wheelchair, or nursing home.

The good news is, you can work to slow and even prevent muscle loss, and the unfortunate ailments that come with it, by exercising to build strength and muscle. And as a study from 2004 in Journal of Musculoskeletal and Neuronal Interactions proves, the sooner you make this a priority, the more you can increase your health span.

> "Physical activity completed when young has residual bone benefits at 94 years of age."

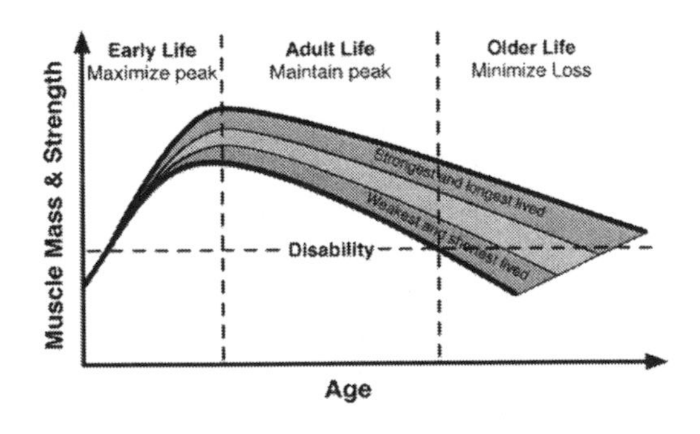

Exercise to Build NOT Burn

When you actually analyze the weight-loss results from exercise, the results are quite depressing. A Cochrane review from 2006 looked at 43 studies on exercise and weight loss, with time periods ranging from 3-12 months, frequencies of 3-5 times per week, and an average workout time of 45 minutes. The average weight loss?

2 pounds!! Generally speaking, this is because exercise (at least when it's in the form of steady-state cardio) creates an energy deficit that's typically filled with more food, and sedentary behaviour.

Sure, it's not about calories-in and calories-out, or strictly bodyweight, but clearly exercising to 'burn' is a poor strategy from the outset. Furthermore, the distances and frequencies most 'exercise-burners' and competitive runners, cyclists, and swimmers take part in, generate unhealthy amounts of cortisol, lactate, free radicals, and inflammation. Which as discussed in *Eat Meat And Stop Jogging*, this creates a high-fat, low muscle, metabolically inactive physique, that's essentially wearing down from the inside out.

The small but critical mind-shift that needs to take place is that we're not exercising to LOSE (as we're already shedding body fat with our efforts in the kitchen), we're exercising to GAIN! A longer, stronger, disease-free life.

The focus of *1% Fitness* is building and maintaining muscle because individuals that carry more muscle have a higher metabolic rate, lower fat storage rate, and a reduced risk of degenerative disease and mortality.

> Resistance exercise builds fat-free mass, while aerobic (or endurance) exercise burns it.

We are not seeking 'weight loss' through more exercise or less eating, because it doesn't work…and doesn't last! Excess exercise and under-eating equals muscle loss, and this is counter productive.

Eat Your Way to Abs

The fastest way to a flat stomach (without sacrificing your health) is to focus on building muscle that burns fat, and eating in a way that has you burning fat as fuel, instead of sugar. Not only because that's the most efficient use of your time to get the results you desire, but because it gives you the best chance at slowing the aging process; instead of unnecessarily accelerating it.

Those following my *Live It NOT Diet!* plan understand that you can burn fat by eating the right foods, getting adequate sleep, and making a conscious effort to walk more. They've seen the impact that nutrition and lifestyle ALONE can have on their body composition and overall health, and learned that it's possible to burn fat without counting calories, monitoring portion sizes, or exercising 5-6 times/week doing mindless cardio.

Live It NOT Diet! is Step 2 of my 3-step transformation plan. I recommend having a look before getting started, as your nutrition and lifestyle habits are critical to your success with 1% Fitness.

That being said, sarcopenia (muscle loss) is still one of the greatest long-term threats to our ability to remain healthy and function independently as we age, so it's essential that we go beyond diet to prevent it. A great example is a study from 2014, where researchers had men supplement 20g of protein twice per day while one of their limbs was immobile. Despite dietary protein serving as an essential component for building and maintaining muscle, it wasn't enough to slow atrophy in the unused muscle.

Another study from 2010 in the European Journal of Applied Physiology came to the same conclusion. Researchers combined a reduced carbohydrate diet with high-intensity interval sprints, and determined that diet was responsible for fat oxidation and insulin sensitivity, while exercise supplied no additional fat-burning benefit, but helped preserve lean muscle mass.

So, even though you can reprogram your body to burn fat with very little training, the 14 nutrition and lifestyle principles in *Live It NOT Diet!* don't quite provide all the necessary support.

Going forward, you can think of it like this:

> Exercise is necessary for building and maintaining strength and muscle, while nutrition is the key to fat loss and metabolic health.

1% Fitness

When we combine the nutrition and lifestyle principles outlined in *Live It NOT Diet!* with the *1% Fitness* principles you're about to read, we put our best foot forward in postponing disability and prolonging vitality. Other than the prevention of muscle loss (sarcopenia), the combination of resistance training and a proper nutrition plan reduces your risk of degenerative disease (heart disease, diabetes, osteoporosis, etc.) and has the potential to reverse what's often referred to as the 'Biological Deterioration Process':

- Insulin resistance
- Strength reduction
- Metabolism slowdown

Provided you're already following the *Live It NOT Diet!* nutrition and lifestyle principles, *1% Fitness* asks for less than 100.8 minutes of your week (10,080min in a week*1%). Leaving you with plenty of time to concentrate on more important activities, like spending time with family and friends, excelling at your career, discovering a new hobby, or simply 'maxin and relaxin;'

> When you spend the limited time you have available to exercise (100min) focusing on building muscle, you burn more fat in the remaining 9,980min a week.

As you'll discover, the optimal fitness approach encompasses brief resistance training (weight-training) routines that stress large muscle groups for multiple sets. Not only because it's highly efficient, but because it produces more metabolically active muscle, burns more fat, and raises critical muscle building hormones; without the elevated stress, excess lactate, and free radical damage characteristic of exercising to burn.

For those that are reading this and feeling intimidated, don't! As the training level you start with has nothing to do with where you'll end up. Police officers, accountants, civil servants, stay-at-home moms, realtors, lawyers, technology gurus, financial advisors, and former athletes just like you have been hugely successful following the principles laid out in *1% Fitness*.

The philosophy is simple:

"Be Better Today Than Yesterday."

And so is the plan:

- Feed the Muscle and Starve the Fat in the kitchen (*Live It NOT Diet!*)
- Build the Muscle that Burns the Fat in the weight room (*1% Fitness*)

1% Fitness is the exact progressive approach I've perfected with my personal clients to help them transform into lean, strong, healthy, athletic machines. It's the culmination of 15 years of personal experience and self-study designed to bring you the optimal solution for transforming your body and improving your life without spending hours in the gym.

I hope you will join me!

Coach Mike

"Even our most highly trained athletes pale in comparison to these ancestors of ours... We're certainly weaker than we used to be."

— Dr. Colin Shaw

PRINCIPLE #1

Mimic Ancestral Movement

Despite a few minor adaptations, we are nearly identical to our ancestors that walked the earth over a million years ago

> 99.5% of our genetic makeup mirrors a human being that relied on hunting and gathering to survive.

Yet, as we discussed in *Live It NOT Diet!*, our diet and lifestyle is not. Largely because we're exposed to a very different daily environment, filled with very different stressors, but also because hunter-gatherers were consistently active

The majority of this physical behavior consisted of low-intensity movement (walking upwards of 5 miles per day on average), that was often times weight-bearing (because of the need to carry food, supplies, tools, and even children). When hunter-gatherers weren't walking and carrying, they were regularly crouching, climbing, bending and lifting. And at times, they also engaged in more intense movement like jumping, running, and throwing; but this was usually while hunting, being hunted, or playing.

A group of researchers in a 2011 study in Progress in Cardiovascular Disease define this type of activity as 'organic fitness,' or 'cross training' and believe it's: *"ideal for developing and maintaining fitness and general health while reducing risk of injury."*

Unfortunately, with each new advancement (agricultural, industrial, and technological revolution) we've become more sedentary, and increased the discrepancy with our highly active genetic makeup. Now, we're exposed to less outdoor activity, more chronic stress, and less time to relax, play, and be social. And as the evidence suggests, this lack of daily movement, combined with an agriculturally dominated, highly processed diet, is why we're experiencing widespread disease.

> Several large population-based studies in U.S., Canada, and the U.K. have determined that only 15-20% of the adult population gets the recommended 150 minutes of physical activity per week.

Along with moving a lot less than the hunter-gatherer, we move a lot differently. For instance, when's the last time you sat like this:

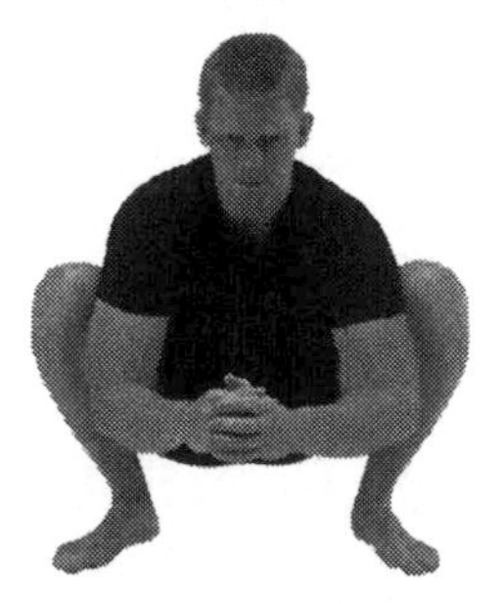

Not only do you frequently sit at a desk or on a couch, but you probably haven't sat in a deep squat since you were a baby. Likewise, you probably sit in a chair on your way to work, instead of walking there.

> In North America, we sit in a car to get to a desk chair, where we'll remain for 8hrs. Then we'll sit in a car to get to a couch, until it's time to lie down for 8hrs.

I get it. That was then, and this is now. We've made advances in technology that have improved our lives by keeping us warm, safe, and comfortable. The point is, we rarely perform the natural bodyweight movements that used to be attempted regularly. Chairs, computers, cars, and shoes have produced a weak, deformed, immobile frame that struggles to execute these basic maneuverers without discomfort.

Obviously, you're not going to quit your job, sell your car, and become a Bushman, but there's no reason why you can't do your best to follow an exercise and lifestyle plan that mimics ancestral living.

Who says you have to sit at work?

Who says you can't walk to the grocery store?

Who says you need to wear high heels or uncomfortable dress shoes?

These may seem like small changes, but they are the same small changes that have created the guy who can't squat, the girl with back pain, and the population where obesity and diabetes are expected.

STEP 1 – WALK & SQUAT MORE

There should be no need to discuss walking, as Principle #10 in *Live It Not Diet!* has you performing 30 minutes of leisurely low-intensity movement every day. But for those that missed it, or can't remember why they're walking, here's a brief summary of the major points.

The average North American may perform 5,000 steps day, but we're designed to be performing more than twice that (5 miles or 10,000 steps per day).

> In 2010, the ongoing Japanese Nakanojo Study determined that the optimal threshold for improved physical health is greater than 8,000 steps/day!

Regardless of our environment, we're genetically predisposed to perform an extremely large volume of daily physical activity. This substantially alters the expression of a significant number of genes related to heart health, immunity, glucose management, and a variety of other key factors.

"Walking is a man's best medicine."

The main reason for walking daily is to prevent disease and mortality. Research has shown its effectiveness in reducing blood pressure and inflammation, improving memory and cognitive function, and increasing lifespan. However, we can also expect modest improvements in body composition because of increases in fat burning, improvements in insulin sensitivity and reductions in cortisol.

> Researchers in the journal Medicine and Science in Sports and Exercise, published a study in 2012 that had regularly active people (nearly 13,000 steps per day), reduce their activity per day to less than 5,000 steps. In only 3 days they decreased their insulin sensitivity by 30%!

Fat is not only the predominant fuel source during lower-intensity exercise, but research points to superior fat loss with higher exercise 'frequencies' as opposed to 'durations.' Meaning, the more 'often' you move, the better results; and with a low-impact, low-intensity, stress-reducing exercise like walking, performing it regularly is very feasible.

One of the driving forces in the health improvements from walking are because of its ability to reduce inflammation. Similar to our anti-inflammatory eating strategy, this anti-inflammatory exercise is a significant contributor to the health of our brain and heart, and overall longevity.

> Just 20 minutes of walking reduces hypertension by 29%, and improves brain function by 1800%!

Walking's impact on the brain appears to be the most impressive. As along with reduction inflammation, it supports the function of brain neurons; which leads to improved memory, mood, and cognitive function, and a lower risk of dementia and depression.

> One 2012 study from the journal Neurology, looked at elderly adults and determined that those who were least active had a 230% greater risk of Alzheimer's, than those that were the most.

In a similar study:

> Harvard researchers found that the brains of those who do regular physical activity have a 20% lower risk of cognitive decline, and are equivalent to being 3 years younger.

Since cognitive function is known to be an independent predictor of morbidity and mortality in the elderly, walking becomes an integral component to extending our health span.

Regular activity also has a positive impact on AGEs (Advanced Glycation End Products), which are a key risk factor for heart disease, dementia, and diabetes. Specifically, it's been shown to lower Hemoglobin A1C (the AGEs biomarker) more than many diabetes medications:

> A 2010 study on 70 participants with Type 2 Diabetes determined that the group exercising 3 times a week dropped their A1C score by 0.73, whereas a sedentary group increased their A1C score by 0.28.

As you learned in *Eat Meat And Stop Jogging*, chronically elevated blood sugar (hyperglycemia) is a common theme in degenerative diseases of the brain and heart, and it's largely driven by a reduction in glucose tolerance (insulin resistance). One of the reasons we see such drastic improvements in disease prevention with walking is because it improves our sensitivity to insulin and helps normalize blood glucose.

In the Diabetes Prevention Program, researchers determined that 150 minutes of walking per week reduces type 2 diabetes risk by 58%!

Since, impaired glucose tolerance is also associated with cancer, this is likely why we see walking correlated with cancer reduction.

The American Cancer Society Prevention Study II Nutrition Cohort collected data from 73,615 postmenopausal women and found that those walking more than 7hrs per week had a 14% lower risk of breast cancer than those walking less than 3hrs.

The best part about all these improvements in health is that they don't require much effort (or cost). You can significantly reduce your risk without even breaking a sweat. Take the stairs, walk to the grocery store, walk around the mall, do a few laps of the office, putter around while you're on the phone, go for a walk instead of watching TV, walk over to speak to a coworker instead of emailing them, or park your car a little further than you normally do - it's that easy!

Deep Squat Daily

With the convenience that a toilet brings, it's hard to argue that it's even the least bit detrimental to our well-being.

- What used to occur in an unsheltered forest, for all of Mother Nature to witness, now happens in a private room in the convenience of your own home.
- What used to require digging a hole, and maintaining a deep squat for up to a minute, now happens on a comfortable throne that washes your business away with the touch of a button.

Since most of us are going at least once a day (if you're not, please revisit *Live It NOT Diet!*) it's clear that a deep squat is something that used to be performed regularly. In contrast to today, where it's rarely (if ever) executed…

…at least in North America.

Many non-Western cultures still opt for the deep squat as a comfortable sitting position, and some Asian, African, Middle Eastern, and European countries still use 'squat toilets' in their bathroom stalls, as opposed to the conventional variety. One company has even popularized a toilet attachment called 'The Squatty Potty' to mimic the deep squat and create the ideal evacuation angle. And yes, there was even a study testing the amount of strain involved in squatting vs. sitting from the journal Digestive Diseases and Sciences in 2003.

> The squatters' experienced full bowel emptying after a duration of 50 seconds on average, while the sitters reported a 'less satisfactory experience' that took nearly 3 times as long (130 seconds).

Aside from the fact that the toilet is making our elimination experience less than smooth (for lack of a better word); it's making the deep squat feel like a foreign position that's difficult to get in and painful to stay in.

Interestingly, we don't have to look far to see the deep squat performed in North America.

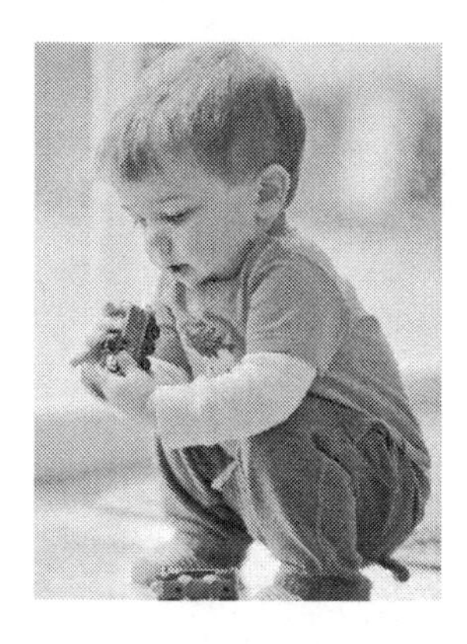

The question is, why does a baby sit comfortably in this position for hours, while the majority of adults fall on their backs, get stuck in the bottom, or can't get into it to begin with?

It's because we don't perform it regularly, so we've lost the ability. Our comfortable chairs, couches, and toilets have made it unnecessary.

But, just like I'm not asking you to quit your job, I'm not telling you to start pooping in your backyard. I'm simply saying you need to start holding a deep squat position for a good amount of time every day.

"Isn't Deep Squatting Bad For Your Knees?"

Other than being aligned with our primitive life, the deep squat is the best way to maintain knee and hip mobility. With research showing that a very high level of knee and hip flexion (165 and 130 degrees, respectively) is necessary to maintain adequate flexibility.

Despite popular belief, research has also proven that there's no difference in stress or force on the knee between squat depths of 70, 90, or 110 degrees. Unfortunately, the original misconception was based on research from 1960 showing an increased prevalence of ligament laxity in deep-squatting Olympic lifters compared to a control group, that was enough evidence for the American Medical Association to advise against squatting below parallel.

Later research was done using the same measurement techniques and showed no such difference. And in fact, the greatest shear force on the knees is when the knees first bend to initiate the squat. Meaning the squat depth is somewhat irrelevant (with respect to the knees), as various studies have shown less force on the AC and PC ligaments at higher knee flexion (i.e. lower squatting depth).

In other words, knee stability is not at risk and there is no 'permanent stretching' of the ligaments taking place at squatting depths below 90 degrees. With some research even finding a protective effect on ligaments from training with higher knee flexion, because of compression of the tissues between the tibia and femur (which rimes them for tolerance to loads in a fully flexed position).

The only way you should be concerned with squatting deep is if you have a previous knee (torn meniscus) or hip problem (cam FAI). For those with healthy knees, squatting deep will only improve their health. In addition to better muscle activation (glutes and hips) and leg hypertrophy, improved functionality in everyday movement, and better athletic performance.

If we return to our discussion from earlier, sitting with fully flexed hips and knees should be a comfortable position for us! It's what we did frequently and effortlessly before couches, cars, and computers.

Executing the Deep Squat Hold

Depending on your current fitness level, getting into the Deep Squat may require a bit of assistance. So, you can use anything from a doorframe to the leg of a table, and don't feel bad about having to hang on for the entire duration (at first).

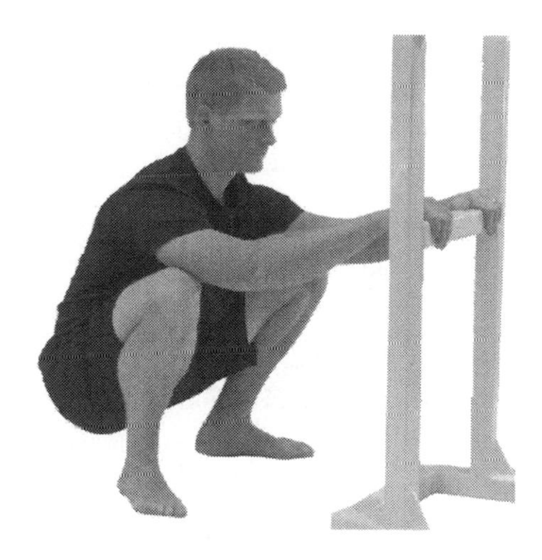

Another option is to perform it on a slightly elevated surface (like a hill or rock), or to elevate your heels (with a wedge or step) until you feel comfortable flat footed.

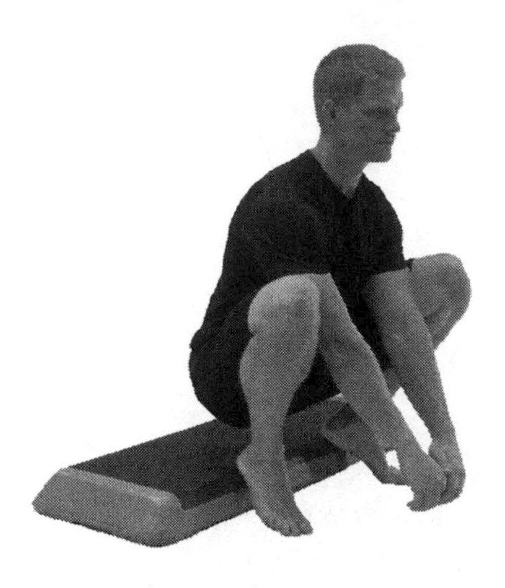

Also worth noting, is that it's okay to round the spine here (as we're not loading it with anything), and moving around and rotating a little is encouraged.

Try starting with 20-30 seconds and look to improve on your time by 5-10 seconds each day. Once you get up to a solid 2-3 minute hold without support, you can start experimenting with multiple sets, or more than 1 deep squat session per day. Since everyone has different schedules, this can be attempted whenever it's convenient. Although, my clients that have had the most success added it before and after their daily walk.

The Deep Squat also serves as a great stretch during the 'Activity Breaks' we'll discuss in Step #2. Trying a Cat Camel (over-arching and over-rounding) maneuver while in the deep squat is recommended for those that have any degree of back pain or strain.

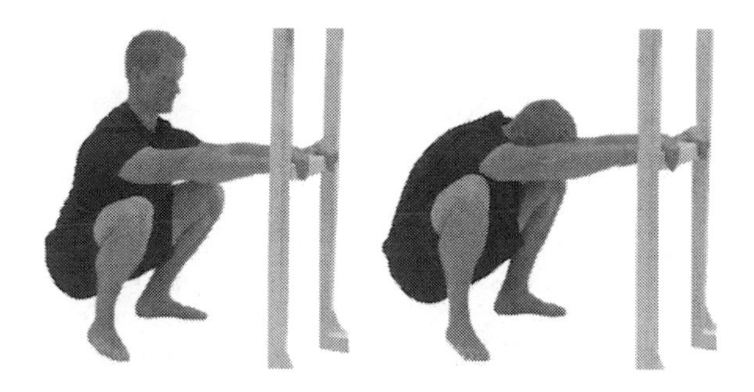

Basically, you perform a Deep Squat Hold while hanging onto a post, and alternate between arching and pulling on the support to draw your shoulders back and chest up, to letting your arms extend and shoulders roll forward while rounding your spine.

Over the years, this exercise has proven extremely useful for providing lower back relief after long days of sitting or standing, and quickly loosening up the hips and knees before weight training.

STEP 2 – SIT & SLOUCH LESS

You've likely already heard that *"Sitting is the new smoking."* And unfortunately, just like smoking, the recommendations to avoid it have taken just as long to surface.

What's worse, is that quitting may be even harder! As there's been a dramatic and consistent rise in sitting time since the 1950's, and it's largely because of inactive transportation, television, and an increase in occupations that revolve around the computer. We sit on the way to work, sit while we're at work, and sit around watching TV when we get home.

Research has demonstrated that approximately 25-35% of adults are inactive, and this sedentary behaviour is a risk factor for heart disease(2.5x), diabetes (2x), and all-cause mortality(0.5x).

> A recent meta-analysis (2015) in the Annals of Internal Medicine reviewed data from 41 studies on sedentary time to find a 91% increase in type 2 diabetes, and 24% increase in all-cause mortality when comparing the most active individuals with the least.

Sadly, it's not as simple as 'more sitting means less moving.' As the research suggests it's the actual act of sitting that's dangerous to our health.

> Evidence from Kansas State University (KSU) in 2013 concluded that those who sit four hours or more each day are at a significantly higher risk of developing cancer, diabetes, and heart disease.
>
> A 2014 study from Northwestern University showed that each additional hour spent sitting doubled disability risk for individuals over 60 years of age.

Both studies found that more exercise didn't counteract excess sitting. Meaning, the person who walks more or spends more time at the gym isn't undoing the time spent at their desk.

Another review from the University of Regensburg in Germany pooled data from 43 studies and over 4 million people to determine that.

> Each additional 2-hour period of sitting per day increased lung cancer by 6%, bowel cancer by 8%, and endometrial cancer (in women) by 10%.

Similar associations have also been made with breast cancer; and unfortunately, the sitting was once again 'independently associated' with the increased risk.

The other important consideration is that the probability of chronic disease remained high regardless of body mass index. Normally, one could argue that those who sit all day have poor eating and lifestyle habits, and this is contributing to the increased risk. However, the evidence clearly demonstrates that the increased risk is not because of the specific lifestyle habits or other outside factors of the individual, but rather the actual practice of sitting. Suggesting that it doesn't matter how lean you are or healthy you eat, you're increasing your risk when you sit too much.

As the lead researcher from Kansas State University Richard Rosenkranz, puts it:

> "We know with very high confidence that more physically active people do better with regard to chronic disease compared with less physically active people, but we should also be looking at reducing sitting."

In other words, we need to make a conscious effort to 'Sit Less.' Not only because more sitting is hurting us, but because more exercise doesn't help.

The only way to avoid the damage from sitting is to not sit!

Stand at Work

If you have a desk job, the obvious solution is designing a workstation that gives you the ability to stand. The adjustable height desk is highly recommended, as it let's you transition between sitting and standing. Plus, it ensures you're able to set a standing height that's aligned with your individual needs (if you share a workstation).

While standing upright with good posture, you should have your:

- Monitor at eye level
- Keyboard slightly below elbow height

After a few days of standing, you're going to notice tired legs and feet. You may also experience pains and strains in new areas, as it's common to over-arch the spine (anterior pelvic tilt), lock out the knees, and favor one hip. This is why it's important to be conscious of your standing position. Not only keeping the head up and shoulders drawn back, but also maintaining a neutral spine, evenly distributing your weight on the 3 pads of your feet, and avoiding favoring one side of the body.

This is also why it's important to take regular activity breaks. As even though standing all-day seems to be better than sitting all-day with respect to energy expenditure, blood flow, and muscle activation, it's also been linked to lower limb problems. Moreover, when research compares a full day of standing to a full day of sitting, the improvements in glycemic control, fat mass, and cardiometabolic risk are minimal at best.

> *Aiming for 10,000 steps before chronically sitting or standing at work for 10hrs is not the same as distributing your 10,000 steps evenly throughout the day.*

Take Activity Breaks

Since not everyone has the luxury of obtaining a treadmill desk, looking to move around every 45-60 minutes appears to be a viable solution for diminishing the damage from chronic sitting or standing. For instance, Australian researchers in a 2013 study from the *American Journal of Clinical Nutrition* had participants complete three 9-hr interventions:

1. *Prolonged sitting* – 9-hrs of sitting, with bathroom breaks when necessary
2. *Prolonged sitting + physical activity* – 15-mins sitting, 30-mins treadmill walk, 8-hrs and 15-mins of prolonged sitting
3. *Regular activity breaks* – 18 x 1-min and 40-sec treadmill walks spaced evenly over 9hrs

Despite taking part in an equivalent amount of exercise (30 minutes total), the activity breaks were more effective at lowering blood glucose (39%) and insulin (26%) than the 'prolonged sitting + physical activity.' Meaning, the person who sits but takes frequent activity breaks is better off than the person that sits for extended periods of time with no breaks, even if they exercise later on.

The best approach appears to be a 5-minute activity or movement break for every 45-60 minutes of sitting or standing. So try setting an alarm on your phone or computer to remind you to walk to the bathroom, grab a coffee, do a lap of the building, or walk over to bug one of your co-workers. Which may seem goofy, but let's face it, so is sitting in front of a TV screen for 8-10hrs a day in a chair.

Stand Tall

Technology is creating a human that's forever slouching. Whether we're rounding our shoulders and back at our desks, or tilting our head to look at our phones and tablets, we seem to be consistently hunched forward. Over time, this produces an extremely poor posture, and muscle imbalances that make us prone to injury. Especially when there's no matched effort to counteract it.

The proper way to stand and walk is with our head up and shoulders drawn back. And we can prevent modern-world damage and improve our posture by practicing this *Active Standing*:

- Drawing your shoulders back by retracting your scapulae
- Straightening your neck by looking straight ahead and tucking your chin

Our hunter-gatherer ancestors probably put a lot less emphasis on it than you'll have to, but they also didn't spend the majority of their lives sitting and hunching.

Chronically hunching over with bad posture is internally rotating your shoulders, which weakens the small muscles of the upper back, and tightens the pecs and shoulders. And since there's no need to hold us upright while sitting, the muscles of the low back and core are also weakening.

World-renowned back expert, Dr. Stu McGill, believes that our desk jobs and sedentary behaviour are to blame for the higher prevalence of *'glute amnesia.'*

Not only are we not using our glutes, but we're losing the ability to properly activate them when we want to. Which is extremely unfortunate, when you understand that they're there to assist and protect other important joints and muscles from damage (like the hips and low back).

Counteract Slouching

Depending on your job and total desk time per day, you may want to consider a few activation and mobility exercises after long periods of sitting or standing. The original versions of these exercises were designed for the gym, so they've been revised for the cubicle:

Standing Cat Camel (+Glute Squeeze) - Alternate between arching your back (by sticking your butt out) and rounding your spine (by tucking your butt in). For additional glute activation, clench or squeeze your butt when you tuck your spine in and hold for 5seconds. Repeat for 5-10 reps.

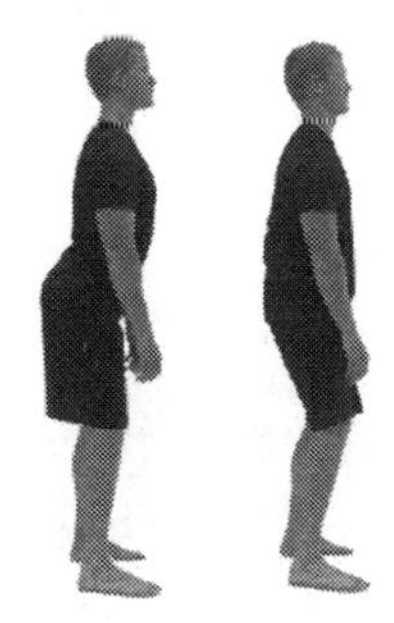

Bent-Over Arm Raises (Thumbs Up!) - Bend at waist to stretch the hamstrings, and go through the following 2 moves with your arms. Repeat for 5-10 reps.

- *Lateral Raises* – with thumbs up and turned back, bring your arms out to the side and raise them as high as possible.

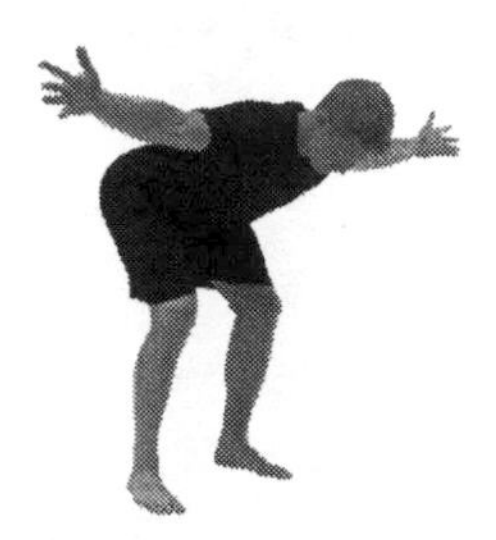

- *Front Raises* – with thumbs up and turned back, bring your arms forward towards your head and raise them as high as possible.

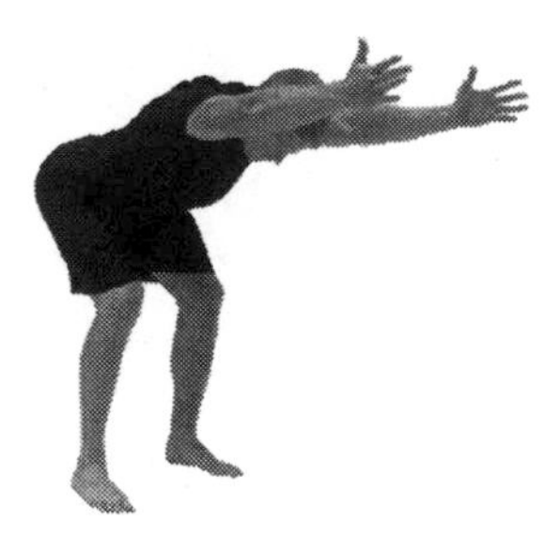

Standing Scarecrow Press – Bring your upper arms (elbow to shoulder) up to parallel with your shoulders and let the lower arm (elbow to wrist) hang to form a 90-degree angle. Maintain the position of your upper arm while externally rotating the shoulder so the hand is now above the elbow as opposed to below, and press the arms straight overhead. Go down the way you came up, and repeat for 5-10 reps.

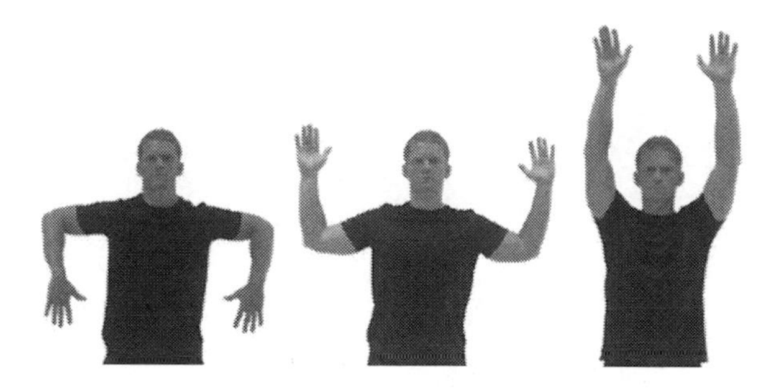

Standing Bent Knee Leg Swings – Position yourself beside a desk or post, hanging on with the hand closest to the support. Swing the same side leg front to back, seeking height with the knee and heel, and maintaining an upright upper body. Repeat for 5-10 reps per leg.

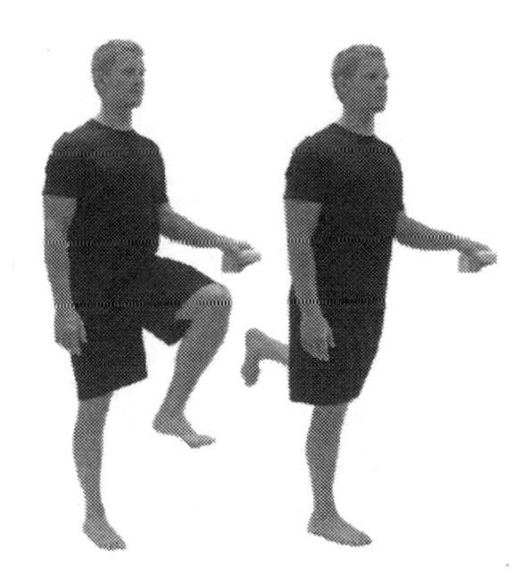

Bent-Over Hamstring Sweeps – Flex your toes towards your shin on one foot and place the heel of that foot 3-6 inches in front of you. While keeping that leg straight reach down towards the floor from as low and far back as possible. Continue to reach while going through a brushing motion towards that foot. Stand, switch feet and continue alternating between legs. Perform 5-10 reps per leg.

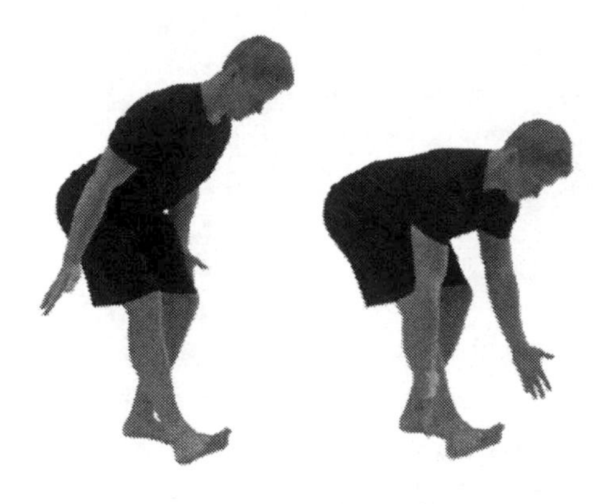

These exercises will help address the tight hip flexors and hamstrings, and underactive glutes, core, and upper back associated with chronic sitting. The 'Deep Squat Hold' is also extremely effective at the office, as it's a great way to counteract the over-arching that can occur when standing for long periods of time, and the tight hips from sitting.

For those that could use a little extra postural work (in addition to their desk drills during activity breaks), look to add a few of these moves to your daily routine.

Cat Camel (All 4's) – Hands Under Shoulders and Hands at Knees

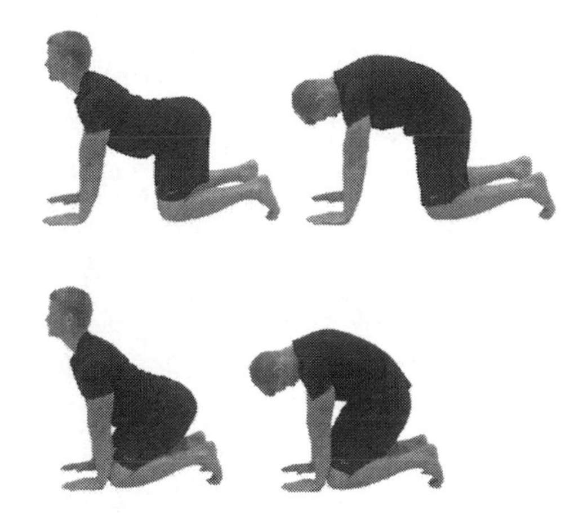

Broomstick Twists – Standing Tall and Bent at Waist

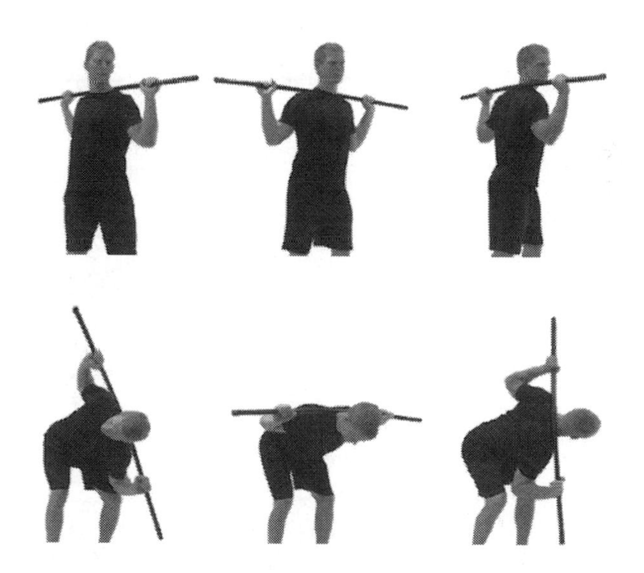

Rubber Band Work – Pull Aparts and Over-the-Tops

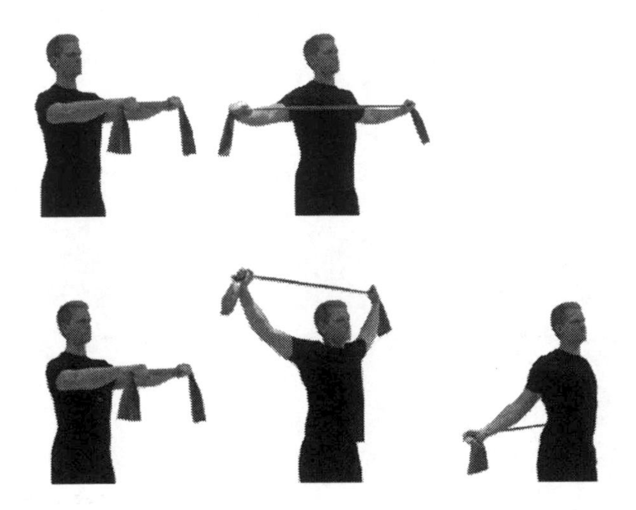

As you'll discover shortly, *1% Fitness* has a dynamic warm-up that's performed before every training session. Some of these moves are executed, but feel free to add any that aren't. Those already dealing with low back/shoulder pain and postural issues, should look to incorporate these into their routine immediately.

Learn to Adapt or Deal With the Consequences

As you attempt to incorporate these habits into your workday, you'll start to notice instances where you sit for no reason when you could be standing and moving around. Phone calls are the perfect example, as the person on the other line doesn't know you're pacing around the office (or playing mini-putt).

The other opportunity is meetings. With 1-on-1 encounters being the easiest, as many times you can go for a walk while talking things through with your colleague. Group meetings may take a little more effort, but that's no reason not to ask (or lie about a bad back like one of my old clients). It simply comes down to how bad you want to get better!

Yes, standing at your desk looks stupid, but so does popping Robaxacet.

Yes, having an alarm go off telling you to move around every hour is disruptive and time-consuming, but so are weekly physio appointments.

Yes, asking your boss to stand in a meeting is somewhat embarrassing, but so is getting wheel chaired into one after knee surgery.

Just like poor nutrition has created your physique, a sedentary life has made you prone to injury. You weren't chosen to live with a bad back, frozen shoulder, or ACL tear, you've consciously made that choice; whether you know it or not.

The question is, what are you willing to do to fix it?

And for those that aren't damaged yet, what are you willing to do to prevent it?

Sitting isn't just messing with your long-term health and body composition, it's making you tight, weak, and deformed. As I mentioned in a Huffington Post article in 2014:

> "You can't out-exercise a crappy diet, and it appears you can't out-exercise a crappy desk job either."

The only way to avoid the detrimental impact of sitting too much is to sit less. So, I suggest figuring out how you're going to make that happen.

STEP 3 – UNLEASH YOUR FEET

The protocol for determining natural movement is pretty straight-forward:

1. Look at hunter-gatherers
2. Look at children

How did we move before technological advances? And how did we move before we were told how to move?

Other than the deep squat reference we just discussed, I used this same illustration to determine whether steady-state cardiovascular training was natural in *Eat Meat And Stop Jogging*. Ultimately discovering that hunter-gatherers ran fast when they needed to (escaping a predator) and children sprinted when they chose to (playing), but otherwise both were consistently moving slow.

They also weren't wearing orthotics, Nike 6.0's, or high heels. With hunter-gatherers going barefoot, protecting their feet with sandals, or wearing a very thin fabric wrap; and babies being born barefoot and usually not wearing anything on their feet until Mom or Grandma takes them shopping. In both cases, this resulted in strong untainted feet that were used as designed - weight evenly distributed on the 3 pads of the foot, significant support from a solid arch, and bones and muscles staying strong because they're consistently loaded.

In the hunter-gatherers case, this is maintained. In the baby's case, it is unfortunately not. Unless of course, the baby is lucky enough to be born into a family that's taken the time to read *1% Fitness.*

> Shoes change the form and function of the foot over time, by providing too much support and permitting unnatural movement.

Why would your arch continue to support when it doesn't have to?

Why would you keep your weight on the balls of your feet, when it's easier to stand flat-footed?

Why would you brace your knees and hips while walking or hiking on a rough surface, when you can wear shoes with built in shock absorbers?

Sadly, you've been wearing shoes for so long, that you've likely never considered how different it feels to walk or run in your bare feet. Generally speaking, it requires a lot more caution and consistent assistance from your knees and hips. Combined with a noticeable transfer of weight from the back of the foot to the front; which is especially evident while walking on a harder surface. The knees need to bend and hips need to sit in order to protect the feet from pain, and the ball of the foot takes control, while the heel seems to barely touch.

Conversely, when your feet are crammed into odd-shaped shoes with an arch support, they conform to an unnatural position, and eventually stop supporting. This not only creates a week arch, but it prevents the flexing and flattening that maintains muscle and mobility.

> "Shoes affect the gait of children. With shoes, children walk faster by taking longer steps with greater ankle and knee motion and increased tibialis anterior activity. Shoes reduce foot motion and increase the support phases of the gait cycle." Journal of Foot and Ankle Research, 2011

The Foot is the Shoe

We are not born with shoes, so we rely on our feet for support. Fortunately, they are designed to withstand all of the walking, sprinting, standing, and jumping we decide to put them through.

In fact, the muscles in our feet (there are over 20) get stronger the more they are stressed. So, if we're consistently walking barefoot, they get used to providing arch support on a daily basis. Whereas, if we're frequently walking in shoes with an arch support, they get used to doing nothing.

> In 1995, researchers in the Journal of Bone & Joint Surgery determined that flat feet were more common in children that wore shoes before the age of six (8.2%), compared to those that wore none (2.8%). The development of the longitudinal arches in the bare footers was also significantly greater overall.

Many are surprised to learn that our feet are designed to grab the ground and assume the surface they're walking on. As depicted in the American Journal of Orthopedic Surgery in 1905, this is how your feet would look if you never put them in shoes.

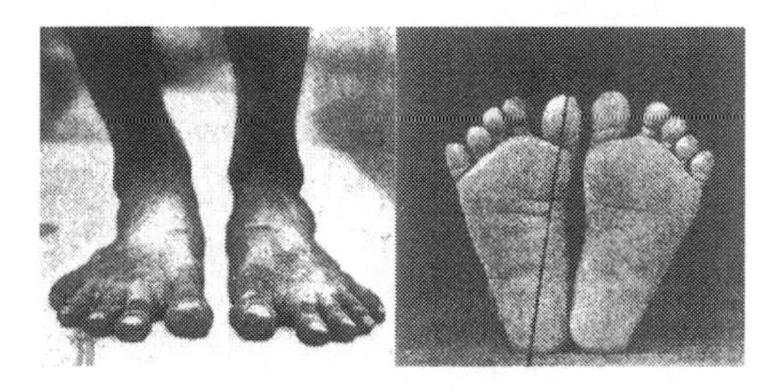

Dr. Philip Hoffman, the orthopaedist that delivered this "Comparative Study of Barefooted and Shoe-Wearing Peoples," also included this fantastic visual to show the deformity that occurs from shoes:

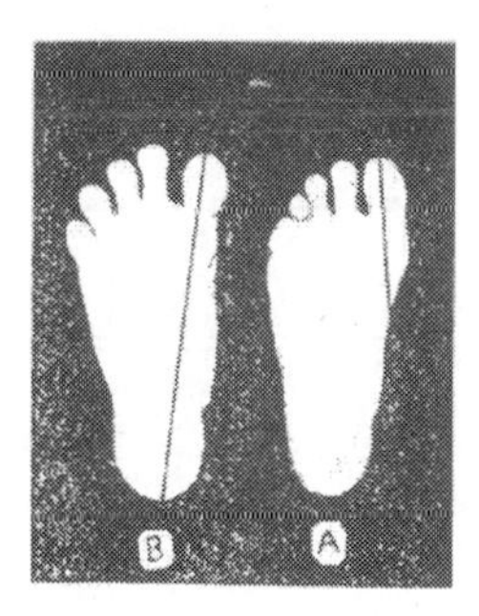

The foot on the right (A), is a child's foot after 3 months of wearing shoes. And the foot on the left (B) is an adult's foot after a lifetime of going barefoot. Yet the toes in foot A are already starting to curl, and the big toe is angling inward.

Interestingly, it's been suggested that the impact of shoes on our feet is comparable to wearing restrictive mittens that didn't allow you to make a fist. With the feet experiencing the same dexterity loss that would be felt in the fingers, and the noticeable discomfort in the wrists, forearms and shoulders.

The difference being, your feet are supporting your entire body!

Similar to any structure, when you weaken the base, the parts above shift and adjust to compensate. Thus, when we lose the strength and change the shape of our feet (the base), the way our hips and knees align, and how the muscles fire to hold our weight changes. Which may not be felt overnight or obvious right away, but will eventually result in pain and deformity in the knees, back, and feet, from the chronic restriction and compensation.

The sad part is, as your feet get weaker and discomfort continues, the more supportive shoes and orthotics you'll seek. Meaning, weaker and more deformed feet over time.

Rebuild Your Arches

Your arches are designed for consistent muscle tension when you're on your feet. This tension holds your arches up and your foot bones together. The more the arch is asked to support, the stronger it gets. The less the arch needs to support, or when it has a consistent supportive system doing the work for it, the weaker it gets.

> Fail to consistently challenge your feet, and the muscles will weaken. Fail to work them at all, and the muscles will atrophy.

Again, the answer is not quit your job and move to the woods to please your feet. It's coming up with a strategy to do the best you can in the circumstances you're given. Here are some ways you can do that with your feet:

Go Barefoot When Possible – In your home, at the cottage, or at a park. Practice walking in bare feet for short stints outdoors, like watering the grass or going to get the mail.

Improve Foot Mobility - Point and flex at full ranges (toes & ankles). Spread your toes and rotate your ankles. Get used to moving your feet around more.

Increase Foot Strength

- *Invisible High-Heels* - Stand and walk on tippy-toes
- *Flex to Point* – Move from heel with dorsiflexed foot (toes up) to ball with full point
- *Angled Toe Points* - Transition from flat foot to balls of feet at various angles and various surfaces (ex: stair) for multiple reps.
- *Side Rolls* – Roll from outside edge of foot to ball of foot with full point of toe
- *Bounce Walks* – Walk forward on balls of feet, while bouncing from low heel (1 inch from ground) to high heel
- *1-Foot Balance & Grab* – Balance on front pad of 1 foot, while trying to grab floor with toes.
- *Sand Walking* – If you have the luxury

Note: *Google 'Coach Mike's Foot Rebuilding Video' for a demo*

Purchase Minimalist Shoes (Vivo, Vibram, etc.)

- Look for wide toe box, flexible sole, no drop (heel and toe same height), minimal-to-no cushion and ankle support
- Start with standing and short walks until your feet build up a baseline of strength
- Practice standing and walking on the balls of your feet
- Avoid running or sprinting until you have been walking for a considerable number of weeks (4+) without soreness.

Word of caution, is that there's a high likelihood your physio, doctor, or orthoepedic salesman will call me a quack, and you an idiot. When this happens, I suggest proving your point by asking them to take off their shoes and walk across the room on the balls of their feet.

Realistically, anyone that's been wearing orthotics their whole life is not a foot expert; and anyone that makes a living off treating your bad feet is not interested in strengthening them. I say this with a bit of frustration because when I was 15 years old I went to see a renowned foot specialist for orthotics, who said it was 'weird' that my toes gripped the ground when balancing on 1 foot.

> Our feet continue to weaken with each new day in shoes; and this is true whether you're the 20% that's already flat-footed, or the 79.9% that's going to be.

There's no guarantee that going barefoot can reverse your fallen arches or flat feet, but there's plenty of success stories of individuals improving the performance and function of their feet. Whether your arches return doesn't change the fact that you're strengthening some of the most important muscles in your body, and giving yourself the best chance for improvement.

> "Nearly 25% of the bones and muscles in your body are below the ankle"

Shoes are essentially coffins for your feet, and the rebuilding program I've outlined above is what needs to be done to bring them back to life. You truly have to work at strengthening your feet, and unfortunately they will be noticeably sore and tired throughout the process. Don't panic when your arches feel like they're going to burst after a 10-min stroll in your new minimalist shoes; and don't think that you can all of a sudden go for a barefoot sprint on your first day. Currently, your feet are a deformed little baby, so we need to teach them how to crawl first!

"Let us bust the myth of physical activity and obesity. You cannot outrun a bad diet."

— Dr. Aseem Malholtra

PRINCIPLE #2

Workout to Build Not Burn

For whatever reason, there's still a general consensus that cardiovascular fitness is the key to longevity. Perhaps it has something to do with cardio burning calories, and an overall deficit promoting longevity?

Well, aside from it being extremely difficult to reach a caloric-deficit via exercise, research suggests that any excessive output is usually filled with more food, and tends to promote an increase in sedentary behaviour. Moreover, going faster, further, and more frequently in an effort to 'burn,' actually damages your long-term health. Because, as we discussed in *Eat Meat And Stop Jogging*, this behavior produces excess cortisol, free radicals, and inflammation; which increase our risk of degenerative disease and mortality.

The other reason it's common to think cardio is best for longevity is because it improves our aerobic capacity. Meanwhile, this is an inferior biomarker for longevity that reduces the superior biomarkers when it's actively and consistently pursued.

Predominantly because excess endurance exercise produces a poor Testosterone-to-Cortisol ratio and a shift in muscle fiber type (Type II to Type 1), that results in the same muscle loss experienced with aging.

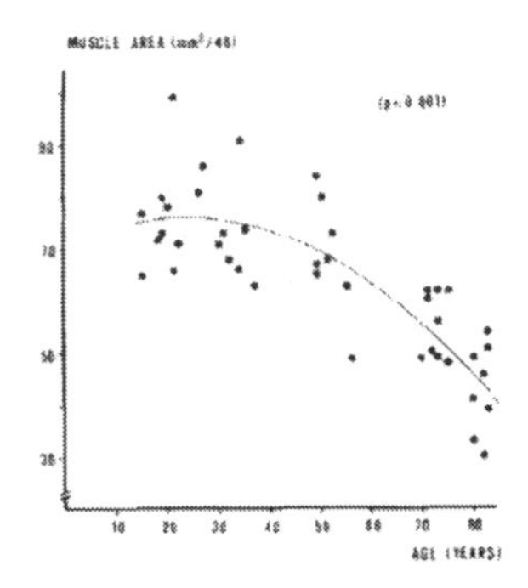

Low Muscle = High Mortality

For the 90 million Americans that will be over 65 years of age by 2050 this is usually an eye opener, but it should be a wake up call for all age groups. As muscle atrophy (loss) starts at the age of 25, and accelerates rapidly if there's no effort to prevent it.

The leg scans below show the impact from a lack of muscle (dark area) maintenance, and the consistent conversion to fat (white area) over time.

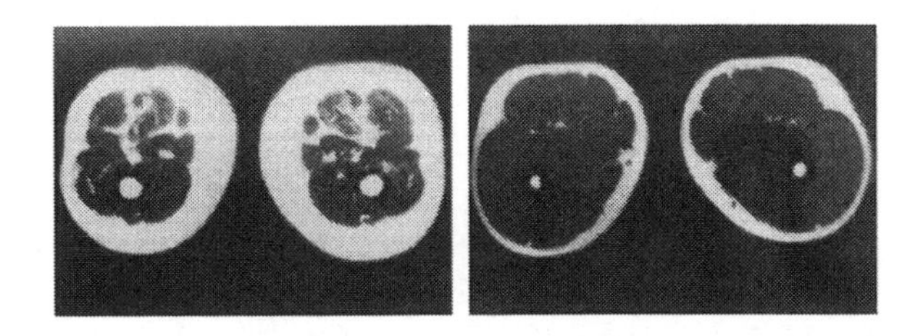

Had the older woman in the scan on the left prioritized strength training when she was a younger woman (the scan on the right), this could have been prevented. Instead, she'll deal with a weak, frail body that's prone to falls, fractures and chronic disease. She'll also struggle with weight management, as this low-muscle physique means a reduced metabolic rate and poor insulin sensitivity. Not only producing a high-fat physique, but raising ones risk of type 2 diabetes, heart disease, dementia (cognitive decline), and even cancer.

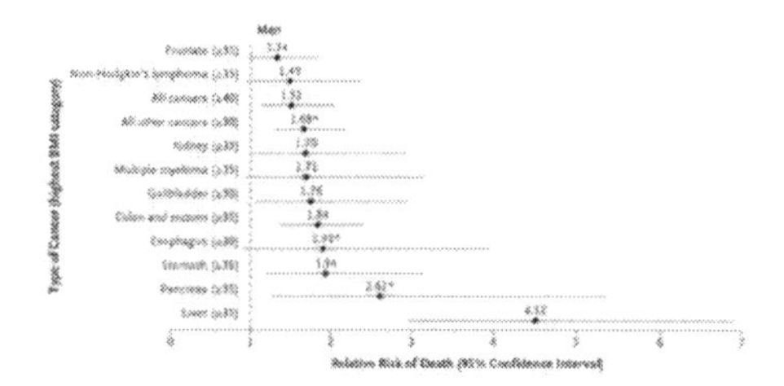

Also worth noting, is that the decline in muscle strength is not only the result of sarcopenia (loss of muscle mass), but it's because of selective atrophy of the explosive or fast-twitch type II muscle fibers.

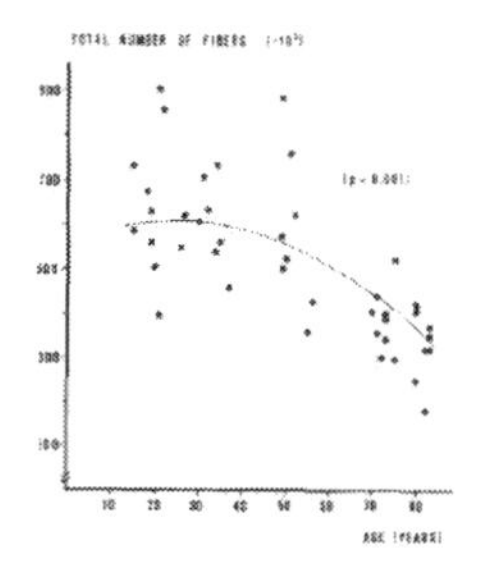

The same muscle fibers sacrificed during aerobic exercise.

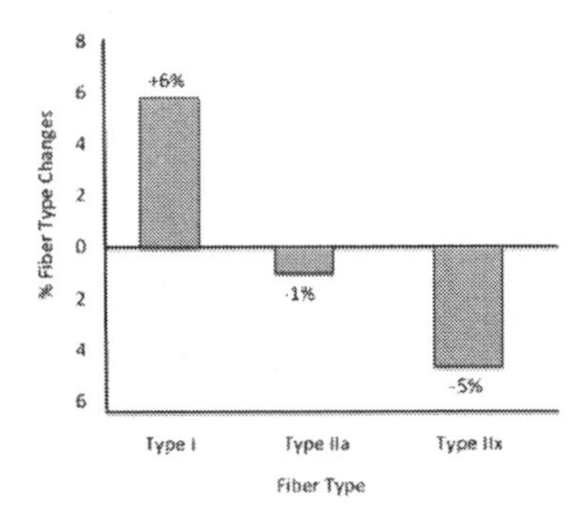

The chart above shows the change in fiber-type after 16 weeks of endurance training.

Alternatively, a fraction of the time spent trying to build aerobic capacity, could have been dedicated to building muscle and strength with resistance training. Preventing the muscle loss associated with aging and increasing strength, insulin sensitivity, metabolic rate, and even aerobic capacity.

The reason aerobic capacity is correlated with muscle loss is because more muscle means more energy producing mitochondria. So when we stress skeletal muscle with weight, it increases mitochondria and elevates it's buffering capacity the same way it does after aerobic training. The difference being, weight training doesn't burn mitochondria-packed muscle; it builds it.

Aerobic training adds mitochondria to existing muscle, while resistance training adds new muscle and increases the mitochondrial number and function of that muscle.

Similarly, improvements in cardiovascular health are commonly credited to aerobic training, even though resistance exercise has the same effect. As this study from 2005 in the Archives of Physical and Medical Rehabilitation demonstrates, strength training (black bars) may actually be superior to endurance training (white bars) when looking at the various heart health markers.

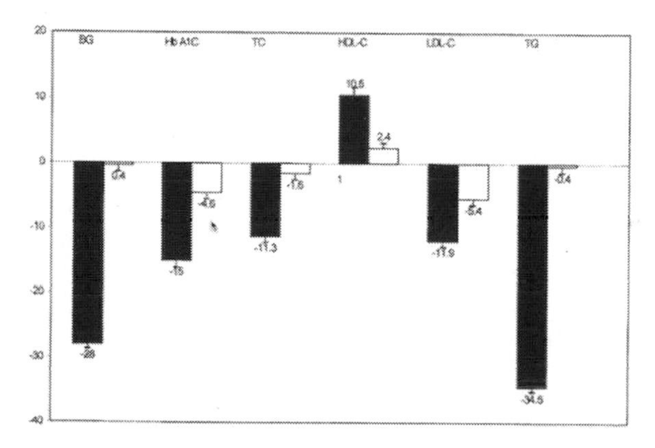

Fig 1. Percentage change in metabolic parameters after 4 months of ST (black) or ET (white). Whiskers represent standard deviation.

Build to Burn

Anaerobic training (weight-lifting or interval training) also burns more calories overall, despite conventional beliefs. Yes, cardio tends to burn more calories during the session, but there's no after-exercise burn, like what's seen after anaerobic-training. Plus, the new muscles built (as opposed to burnt), lead to a higher daily caloric burn going forward.

Since a declining metabolic rate is one of the things that makes weight management difficult with age, we should be dedicating the minimal time we have to exercise towards maintaining or increasing it. Unlike cardio, resistance training elevates this rate (which determines 60-75% of our total energy expenditure) by facilitating muscle maintenance and development.

> "The average middle-aged person's problem is not excess weight as much is it is excess body fat coupled with too little muscle. Simply losing weight is the wrong goal; the key is changing your ratio of body fat (biologically inactive energy storage) to muscle (biologically active tissue). People with a greater ratio of muscle to fat enjoy a higher metabolism and don't have to worry as much about gaining weight or about how much they eat—that active tissue burns more calories." Tufts University

This is likely why a study from 2015 in the journal Obesity, showed twice the reduction in waist circumference for those doing weight training compared to those doing cardio.

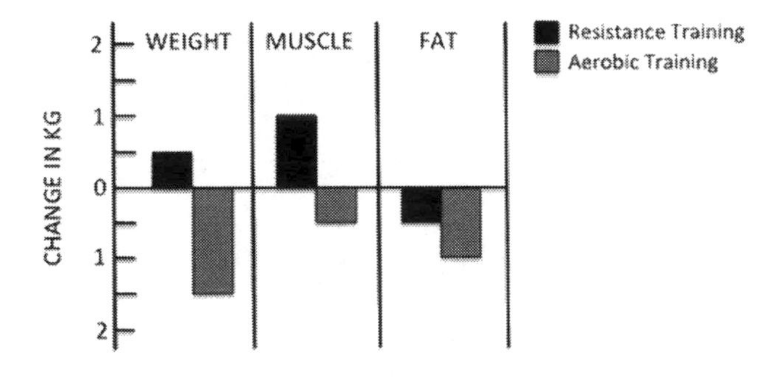

Unfortunately, resistance training's ability to increase lean body mass and burn fat free mass at the same time can discourage those that obsess over the scale. Meanwhile, if they paid more attention to the image in the mirror and the size of their waist, they'd discover how easy it is to get and stay in shape. Because as outlined in the American Journal of Clinical Nutrition in 2006:

> A 10lb increase in lean muscle mass translates to an additional 100kcal of energy output per day, and approximately 4.7kg of fat loss per year.

Lift to Last

Along with building metabolically active muscle and leading to comparable improvements in cardiorespiratory fitness, here is a quick list of some of the additional benefits attributed to resistance training:

- Improves strength and functional ability (in elderly)
- Reduces risk of heart disease
- Increases HDL cholesterol
- Reduces risk of type 2 diabetes
- Prevents osteoporosis (bone loss) and sarcopenia (muscle loss)
- Improves gastrointestinal health
- Burns visceral fat
- Improves glucose tolerance and insulin sensitivity
- Protects against frailty and metabolic syndrome
- Produces metabolic memory and reverses age-related changes in skeletal muscle
- Builds explosive type II muscle fibers (reduced with age)
- Improves dynamic and functional stability (balance) and flexibility
- Increases psychological well being (mood, self esteem) and cognitive function
- Fosters spatial awareness in elderly (less falls)

- Helps control inflammation
- Increases flexibility
- Prevents injuries and disability

Successful aging refers to the maintenance of physical and mental well-being and functional independence in the absence of chronic disease. Resistance training supports this, by upregulating the factors associated with muscle growth, downregulating those associated with muscle loss, and improving muscular power and force development - which research suggests is critical for preserving our quality of life as we age (health span).

Never Too Old

As Irwin. H. Rosenberg stated perfectly in 1997 in his paper on Sarcopenia:

> "No decline with age is as dramatic or potentially more significant than the decline in lean body mass."

Although he was also clear in stating that it wasn't inevitable, and it was never to late. Since the ability to gain and maintain strength and muscle with resistance training is possible whether you're 40, 18, 27, 51, 32, or 90!

As this study from the Journal of the American Medical Association concluded in 1990:

> "Resistance weight training leads to significant gains in muscle strength, size, and functional mobility among frail residents of nursing homes up to 96 years of age."

In other words, regardless of your age, or current health status (insulin resistance, obesity, type 2 diabetes, etc.) there are no non-responders to resistance training. The key is starting as early as you can (Now), and making it into a habit (*1% Fitness*).

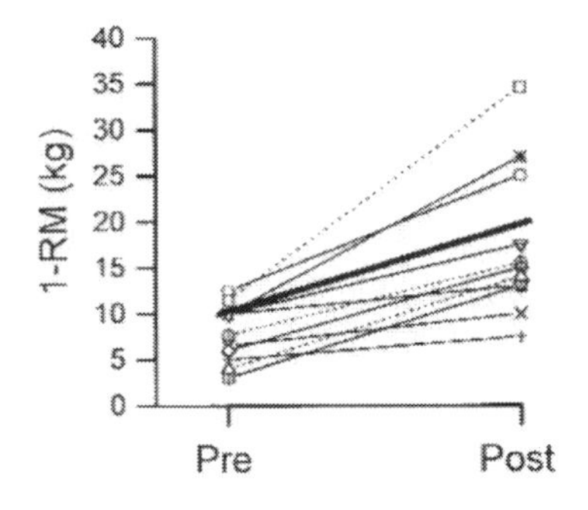

Live It NOT Diet! is already ensuring that your muscle stays fed, and now it's time to make sure it's primed for growth (anabolic). The *1% Fitness* workouts will give you a better looking body with a maxed out metabolic rate, and the best chance at living a long and disease-free life.

Phase 1 – Build a Bodyweight Base

As much as I'd love to fast-track you to the meat and potatoes of *1% Fitness*, it's essential that you successfully execute the bodyweight exercises outlined in Phase 1 at the back of this book. Each bodyweight movement has 4 levels, and I assure you that even the highly experienced will find levels 3 and 4 quite challenging when executed according to the guidelines.

Not only will this introductory phase help prepare your core for weighted resistance, but it will make your stiff, sedentary, computer-jockey life more like your active, mobile, pain-free ancestors. After 2 weeks of building strength and moving comfortably with your own bodyweight, or as I like to call it 'Strong in Your Own Skin,' you'll be introduced to exercises with weighted resistance in Phase 2.

Developing competency in these exercises not only improves your performance today, but it extends into your latter years when it's appreciated most. Aside from the aesthetic reasons, this is why strength and muscle building should be a priority.

Before continuing to Principle #3, flip to the Phase 1 workouts at the back of this book. Along with your effort to 'Mimic Ancestral Movement,' these workouts should precede the weighted resistance in Phases 2 and 3.

"If you think lifting weights is dangerous, try being weak. Being weak is dangerous."

— Bret Contreras

PRINCIPLE #3

Choose Free-Weight Compound Exercises

The term "functional' is often overused, and frequently misused in the fitness industry. However, it's an appropriate word for the type of strength we're looking to build. Essentially, it means getting strong and being strong in movements that are applicable to daily life.

Some would argue that 'all strength' is applicable to daily life, but clearly there are exercises and movements that are more functional than others. For instance, the squat is activating muscles and executing movement patterns that are required to perform the same squatting motion performed in life.

Furthermore, some exercises have a greater return for your investment in time. If you only have 20 minutes to workout, I assure you that your time is better spent squatting than doing bicep curls.

> Squatting is superior for improving movement in everyday life. Bicep curls seem to only be superior for improving ATTENTION in every day life.

Although not all exercises performed in *1% Fitness* are truly 'functional,' they have the highest functional transfer. I'm not one to make excuses, but it's pretty challenging to perform only functional movements with the lifestyle we have, and equipment we have access too. For instance, there's nothing really functional about lying on a bench to press a barbell. However, it's one of the best exercises for building upper body strength and muscle, and is more relevant than isolation or machine exercises.

The best way to think of 'functional' versus 'non-functional' is to put exercises on a continuum.

Standing > Sitting/Lying Down > Machine

Or

Dumbbell > Barbell > Machine

And fortunately, when we prioritize free-weight compound movements, we're always on the upper end of it.

Functional = Free-Weight + Compound

From strictly an efficiency standpoint, it makes more sense to choose compound exercises over isolation exercises because they work multiple muscle groups instead of just one. However, we also select them because they're more relevant to every day life.

Bending, lifting, climbing and carrying is what we're genetically predisposed to execute, and compound movements mimic that environment.

> *Trust me, your hunter-gatherer predecessors didn't spend 2hrs in the gym 6 days a week isolating specific muscle groups to look 'pumped' at the upcoming pig roast.*

Generally speaking, multi-joint or compound movements (like the squat) are best for building functional strength, and single-joint or isolation exercises (like the bicep curl) tend to be 'non-functional.'

The other reason we favor compound or multi-joint movements is because they generate a far bigger hormonal and neurological response. Translating to higher levels of muscle building (hypertrophy) and superior strength development.

The same can be said with respect to choosing free-weights over machines. As a barbell or dumbbell squat is a lot more stressful than a leg press (machine equivalent to the squat), and results in a more significant neurological response when matched for intensity. Not only secreting higher concentrations of muscle and strength building hormones, but promoting faster gains because of the increased adaptations necessary to deal with the stress.

> Research from the 8th International Conference on Strength Training in Norway (2012) compared 6 sets of 8-10 reps in the squat versus the leg press, and found 50% higher testosterone levels, and 3 times the growth hormone for the squatters.

These results are somewhat understandable when comparing compound and isolation exercises, but less straight forward with free-weights and machines. But generally speaking, machines operate in a single plane, whereas free-weights are multi-directional. As if you think of a Seated Shoulder Press Machine - where you can push the handles straight up in one defined direction to lift the stack of weight - your only option at the top is to lower the handles on the same plane or axis that you pressed them, and bring the stack of weight back to it's starting position. Whereas a Seated Dumbbell Shoulder Press, on the other hand, gives you a variety of pressing angles on the way up, and lowering angles on the way down. And although the end result of the exercise may be the same – pushing it straight up, and lowering it straight down – there are more muscles recruited to keep you stabilized with free weights. Since the stabilizer muscles are doing the work that the machine does to keep you on the right path.

It's not that free-weight compound movements are the only way to build muscle, as with the right weight and proper variables (tempo, reps, sets, rest) all exercises can. It's that the exercises that recruit the most motor units produce the best results, and generally speaking, those are the functional exercises aligned with our past.

> Tests have determined that over 200 muscles are activated during the squat.

Best for Injury Prevention

Aside from higher muscle recruitment, neurological responses, hormone secretion, and strength development, free-weights are beneficial for injury prevention. Because unlike machines, they strengthen our stabilizer muscles and familiarize our body with maximal ranges, and a variety of angles.

Life doesn't happen in a single plane, and at times we are challenged in odd and unnatural positions. So, the more comfortable our muscles are through the full range of motion, the lower the probability of a pull, strain, tear, or serious injury. Machine training may accomplish the goal of extending and contracting the muscle, to build some degree of strength, hypertrophy, or muscular endurance, but it's not challenging the body as it's designed to move – as 1 unit!

In fact, one could argue that performing strictly isolation exercises or relying solely on machines could actually increase ones risk of injury, as imbalances put unwanted stress and strain on certain areas. For instance, a big chest without the support from the little stabilizer muscles of the shoulder could result in a shoulder injury while throwing a baseball with some buddies. Or big powerful quads, without equivalent support from the posterior chain (hamstrings, low back, glutes) could mean a pull or tear when going for a short sprint.

Some would say that developing a balanced physique is the biggest reason for prioritizing free-weight compound exercises. Not only for aesthetic reasons, but for injury-free living. Free-weight compound exercises recruit more motor units while strengthening important stabilizer muscles. Mimicking real world performance more than isolation exercises, and developing the functional strength that was characteristic of our ancestors. Sure, you can build chest strength by doing the Seated Chest Press Machine, or quadriceps muscle by using the Seated Leg Extension Machine, but how useful is that in everyday life?

Best for Core

Although you may not realize it, the muscles of your core are constantly working when you're standing upright. And they become more active when you bend to the side or front, carry a heavy bag or object, or need to regain your balance after losing your footing on an uneven surface. This is why our hunter-gatherer ancestors (both male and female) had much stronger and more well-developed core muscles than human beings today.

> Hunter-gatherers weren't just sitting less and walking more, but they were often carrying heavy loads, or doing some form of physically demanding work.

Unfortunately, unless you live on a farm, it's difficult to mimic this type of daily behaviour in our modern environment. And even then, lots of people now 'live on farms,' without having to actually 'work on farms.' In any case, our best chance at developing equivalent core strength is by performing similar work in the weight room.

As you may have guessed, sitting in a chair training 1 isolated muscle group, is not the answer for building a solid core. And this is one of the major reasons isolated machine training should not be prioritized.

In addition to getting far more core activation with a Squat or Overhead Press (free weight compound movements) compared to a Seated Leg Extension or Chest Press (machines), we're mimicking the exercise that's aligned with our high-performing injury-resistant genetics.

Best for Aesthetics

Free-weight compound movements also produce a more aesthetically pleasing physique. Not only because of increased hormonal surges facilitating superior muscle growth, and the support from stabilizer muscles promoting additional development around the primary movers, but because free-weights permit a higher range of motion.

A muscle is at its full range of motion when it's in its fully stretched or contracted position. More stretch and more contraction means more units recruited and greater muscle development. Though not all free-weights allow full range of motion (ex: barbell bench press), they generally provide ranges beyond what a typical machine provides. Moreover, unlike machines, there's usually an alternative (ex: dumbbells) that provides greater range when necessary.

Free-weights also provide the ability to tap into a full range of motion at different angles. For example a Dumbbell Chest Press has various grip and width options, and bench angles. All of them hit the chest and shoulders in a different stretching position at the bottom of the movement, and contraction position at the top.

One could also make a case for the injury prevention that accompanies the elevated range of motion with free weights. Working muscles to their fully stretched position increases their flexibility, and stretching and contracting at a variety of angles familiarizes the muscle with extended ranges. This makes them less prone to a tweak or strain when encountering an over-stretched or over-extended position in every day life.

Although it's typically believed that stretching is the best way to gain flexibility, resistance training is just as effective when performed to full range. These dynamic movements simultaneously improve strength, flexibility, stability, motor control, and muscle development!

"You must do what other don't, to achieve what others won't."

— Henry Rollins

Include the 4 Major Movements (Push, Pull, Bend, Extend)

When looking at hunter-gatherers, the movements involved in daily living included bending, lifting, dragging, carrying, climbing, jumping, and throwing. Although we could execute these exact movements on a daily basis and work to build near-equivalent strength, we need to be realistic in our circumstances. Fortunately, we have resistance training exercises that mimic and strengthen the same muscle groups and firing patterns involved in these maneuvers.

For simplicity, these laborious hunter-gatherer movements have been classified into 4 primary categories that form the backbone of *1% Fitness*:

1. Push
2. Pull
3. Bend
4. Extend

‘Push’ can also be thought of as ‘press.’ It’s any time our hands extend from our body, to push in front of us, overhead, or anywhere in between.

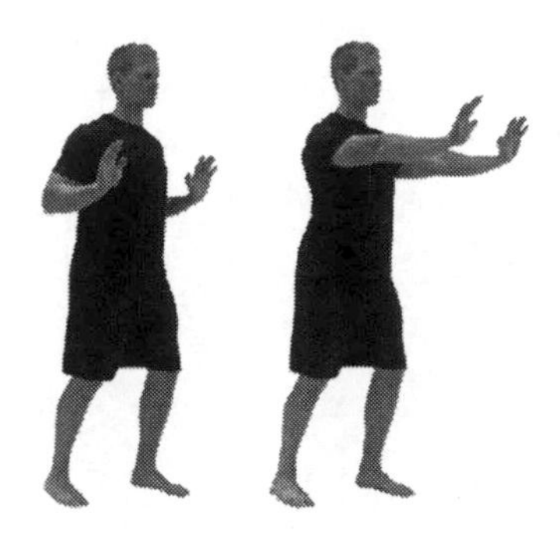

‘Pull’ is to mimic climbing, and it could include any action where the resistance pulls your arms away from your body. In general, this is a pull-down, pull-up or rowing motion.

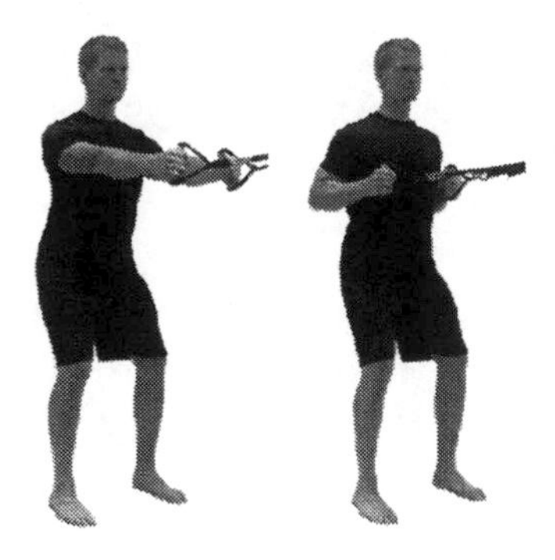

‘Bend’ refers to a knee bend, which you’re already executing daily via the Deep Squat. But additional bending work will be performed during workout times to further develop the strength in our legs and core. The primary bend is the squat, with the lunge not far behind.

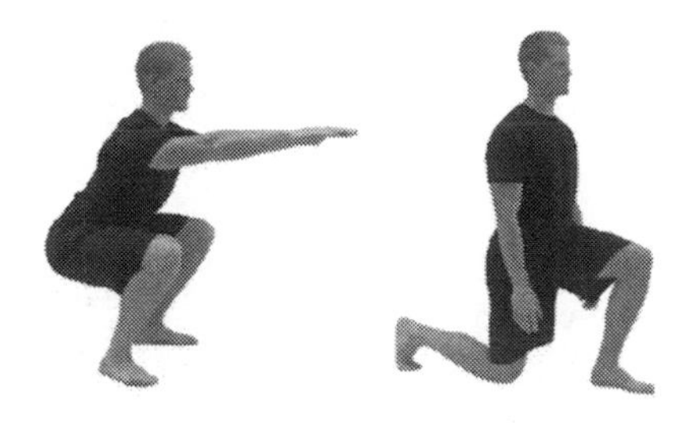

'Extend' is referring to an extension of the hips. Essentially, the hips are back as if we're picking something up, and they come forward when we stand. Along with a knee bend, it's the other action that takes place during a jump; and is often referred to as a hip hinge.

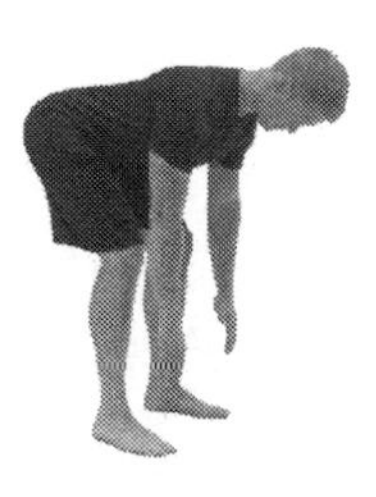

Major Lower Body Movements - Extend

The muscles involved during the different variations of the hip extension exercise (i.e. posterior chain) are very active when squatting or bending to pick things up. These are two movements that were regularly executed by our primal ancestors, and continue to be performed on occasion by you and I (when doing laborious work).

Even if we forget about our DNA, the main reason we should prioritize the hip extension is because it prevents injuries in every day life. Because if you can bend down and pick up your bodyweight with good form, you're not going to hurt your back lifting a 24 pack of water into the car, or bag of yard waste to the end of the street.

> Research from 2011 in the journal Archives of Physical and Medical Rehabilitation determined that the deadlift (standing hip extension) was the most effective exercise for strengthening the paraspinals (lower back), when compared to the back extension, bridge, 1-leg hip hinge, and lunge.

The hip extension (or hip hinge) from a standing position is the main movement involved in a deadlift.

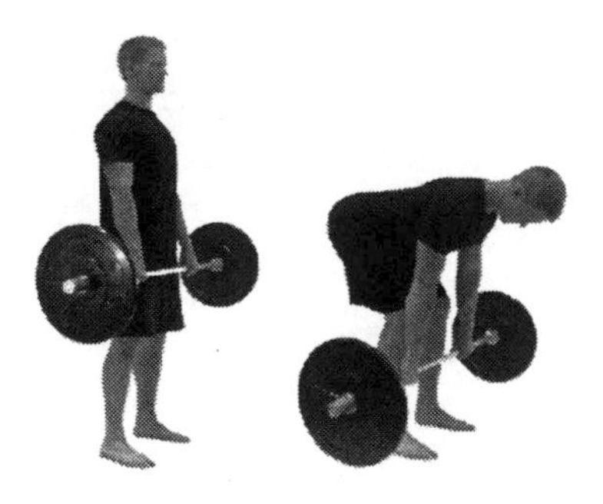

The variation in the picture above is usually referred to as a Straight-Leg, Semi-Stiff or Romanian Deadlift, as opposed to it's Bent-Knee or Standard form with the knees bent.

Unfortunately, the bent-knee version can make things a little complicated with respect to classification, as technically it's a 'Bend' and 'Extend.' Especially when looking at something like a Standard Trap Bar Deadlift:

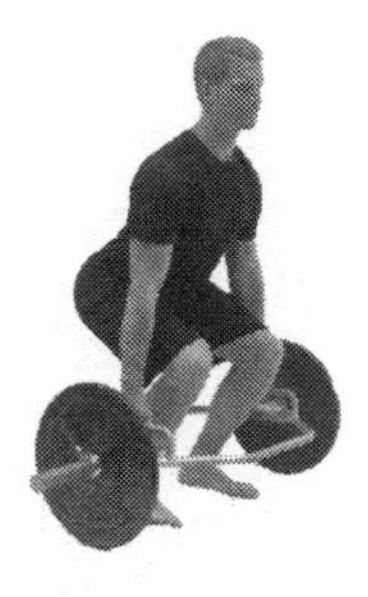

Some would say the exercise in the picture above is a deadlift because you're pulling off the floor, while others would say it's a squat because of the considerable knee-bend and upright torso. But since *1% Fitness* aims to hold true to the 'Bend' and 'Extend' classifications, the Trap Bar maneuver above is a considered a knee-bend. While a hip-extend execution with the Trap Bar would like more like this:

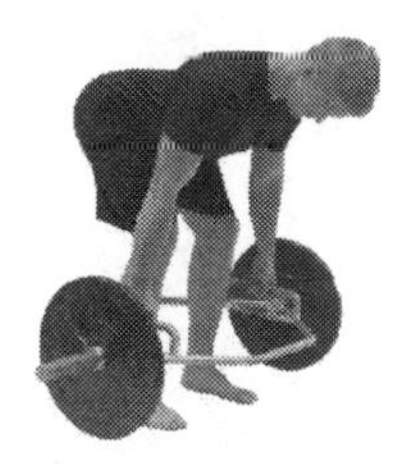

The same principle holds true with respect to the Sumo variations of the deadlift. As depicted in this picture:

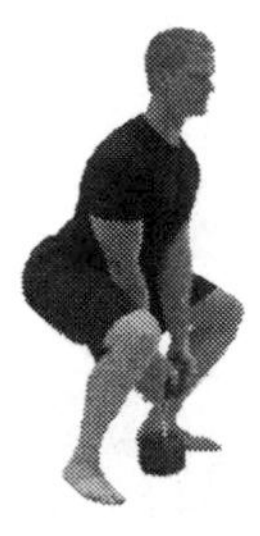

Despite being a pull from the floor, we classify this as a knee-bend because it's more of quad (or anteriorly dominated) exercise, than a hip (or posteriorly dominant) movement. And interestingly, research appears to support that thinking. With a study from 2002 in the journal Medicine & Science in Sports & Exercise showing significantly greater activation in the quadriceps and less in the hamstrings when comparing the sumo deadlift to the standard variation.

The other extension movement you'll come across with *1% Fitness* is the glute bridge or glute thrust, which has been highly-popularized over the last decade by NSCA Certified Strength & Conditioning Coach and Sports Scientist, Bret Contreras. Who teaches us that you can think of the deadlift (or hip hinge) as the ideal movement for the hamstrings, and the Glute Bridge or hip thrust as the ideal movement for the gluteus muscles.

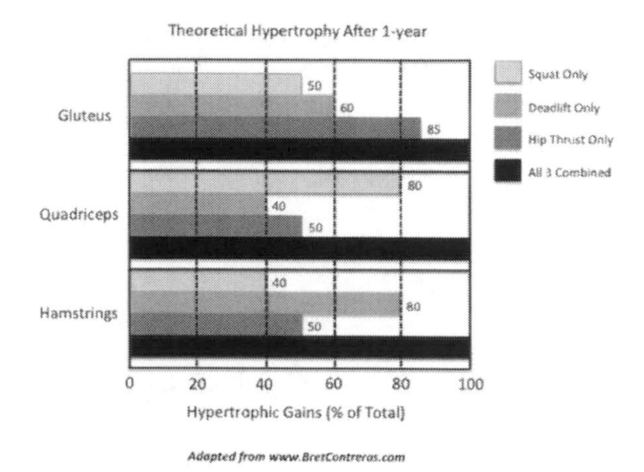

Adapted from www.BretContreras.com

Bret often says the bench-supported bridge's impact on the glutes is comparable to the Flat Barbell Bench Press's impact on the pecs. As both exercises are not necessarily as functional as a standing overhead press or deadlift, but they're extremely effective compound movements for stimulating growth and strength gains in the pecs and glutes.

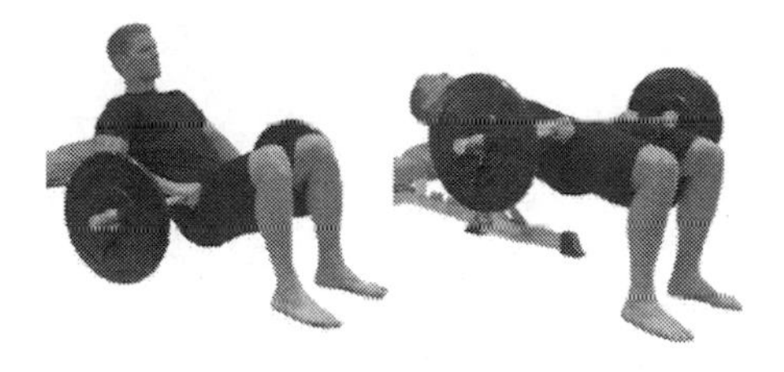

The remainder of the extension movements to be covered in *1% Fitness* are still hip dominant movements, but they focus primarily on the muscles of the lower back. For example, we'll take a look at the Back Extension (or Hyper Extension) at both a 45-degree and 90 degree position.

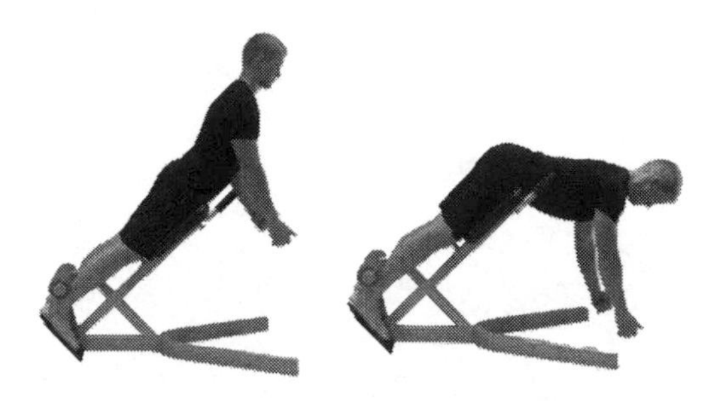

As you'll discover throughout *1% Fitness*, there are a variety of progressive options to make these exercises more challenging and build a stronger low back. Adding weight is the obvious solution, but even something as simple as extending your arms at different times throughout the back extension, make a sizeable difference in difficulty.

Hip Extension Most Important?

Although the Squat (or Bend) tends to be more popular, as the gym rats chase bigger and better quads, the hip extension movement may be more important. Generally speaking, this is because bending and lifting tends to be more common than squatting with a load on our back, whether we're a 2 million year old hunter-gatherer, or a modern-day suburban soccer dad. Sure we bend the knees to lift, but it's predominantly a waist bend.

Additionally, as weights get heavier in knee-bending exercises like the squat, the hips are more heavily recruited than the muscles of the knee. Almost as if naturally our body calls in the big guns (glutes and low back) to handle the increased load. For instance, take a look at the increase in the hip-extend to knee-bend ratio as weights get heavier in the squat:

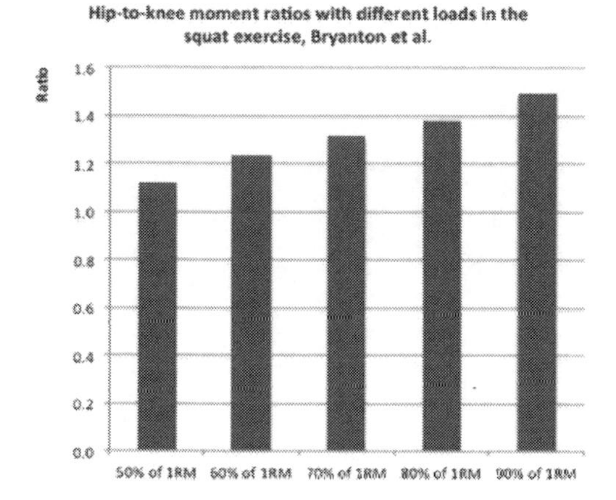

Which we also see in the lunge:

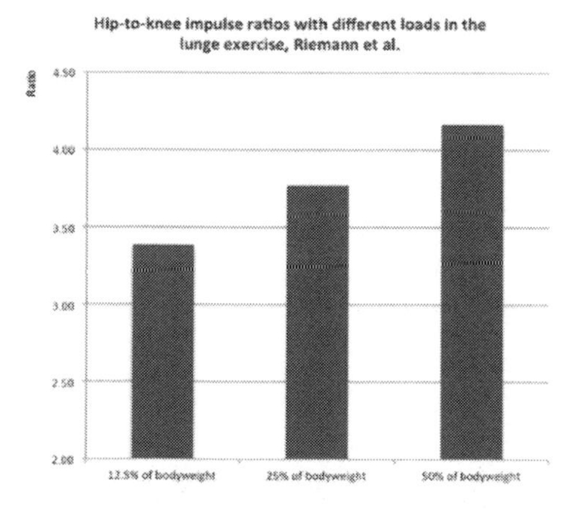

And the traditional (bent-knee) deadlift:

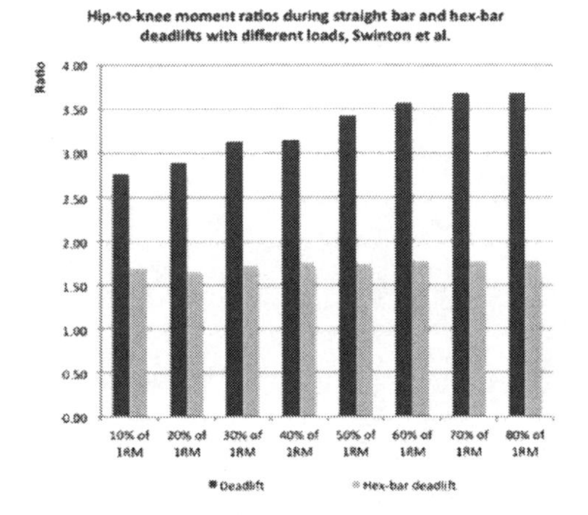

Interestingly, it appears we also look to the hips for more speed and power during dynamic movements. As have a look at the increased contribution of the hips at faster running speeds:

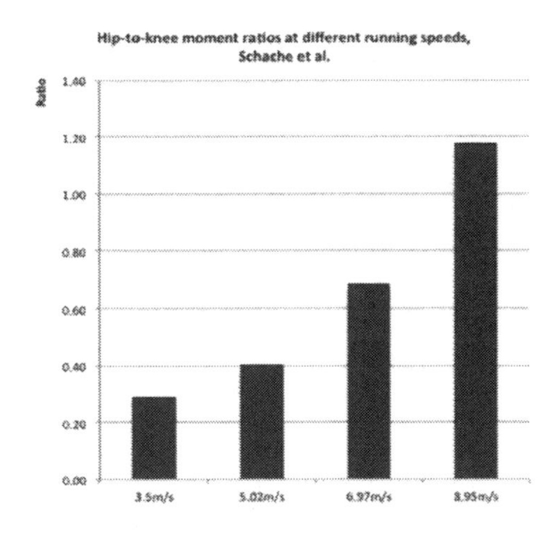

And increased jumping heights:

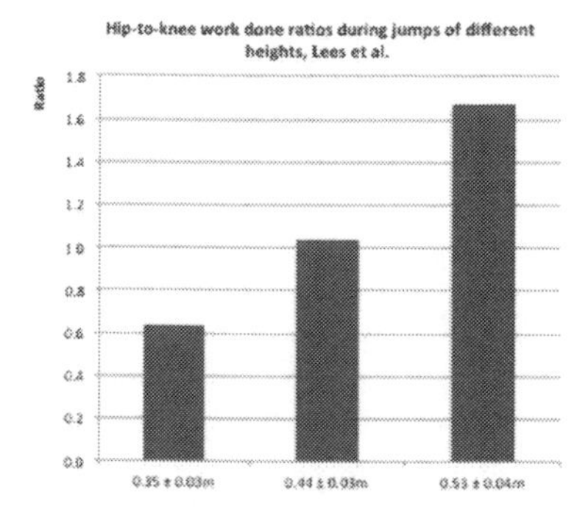

The point is, just because we don't see our backside, doesn't mean it's not worth developing. As far as functional ability goes, it appears the posterior chain and hip extension maneuver is more critical to maximal performance than the quadriceps and knee-bend muscles.

Executing the Hip Hinge

People get hurt in the weight room and in everyday life because they don't know how to pick things up properly. Aside from preventing injuries, repeating and perfecting the hip hinge pattern is critical in teaching you how to stabilize your pelvis and spine. And this grows in importance as we look to progress to more complex (bent-over row) and dynamic (kettlebell swing) movements.

The bodyweight movements in Phase 1 should give you a baseline of strength necessary to feel the muscles involved in the hip hinge, and the beginner variations in the first few workouts of Phase 2 should give you ample opportunity to practice. However, this can be a challenging maneuver for many to perfect at first; which is why the Butt-to-Wall drill can be quite useful for improving body awareness and overall technique before loading the movement.

Butt-to-Wall Drill – With your back towards the wall, position your heels approximately 1 foot away. Stand up straight with your hands on your thighs. Set an arch in your back by poking your butt up (like a cat in the cat camel) and puffing your chest. With slightly bent knees (10-15 degrees), start to bring your hands down your quads while pushing your butt towards the wall. When your butt touches, return to standing while maintaining your posture. Look to increase your distance from the wall until you reach a point where you feel a hamstring stretch before your butt touches. That hamstring stretch is as far as you want to go with your weighted hip hinge. If you're reaching the floor before getting a hamstring stretch, you need to fix your posture; try performing the exercise in front of a mirror.

Major Lower Body Movements – Bend

The predominant knee-bending activity in *1% Fitness* is the squat. As discussed earlier, this would've been a regular movement in everyday living to scavenge, build a fire, and go #2 in the bush. It's also the other primary action (with hip extend) involved in picking something up, jumping, and running - movements that were necessary for our primal ancestors to survive, and movements that are required to live a long and disease-free life today.

> "The squat movement pattern is arguably one of the most critical fundamental movements necessary to improve sport performance, to reduce injury risk, and to support lifelong physical activity."
> *NSCAs Strength & Conditioning Journal, 2014*

Although there are various ways to teach and execute the squat based on your training goals (bodybuilder, powerlifter, athlete, etc.), there are commonalities in all forms that produce considerable increases in physical attributes, and injury reduction. With the Barbell Back Squat being the most well-recognized, and often regarded as the most effective way to enhance the explosive movements necessary to excel in athletic performance.

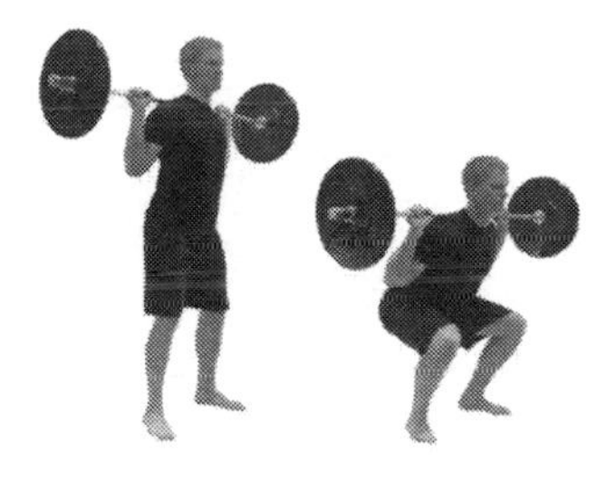

However, similar to the hip extension, there are a variety of ways to load and execute the squat that are equally challenging and effective in their own unique way.

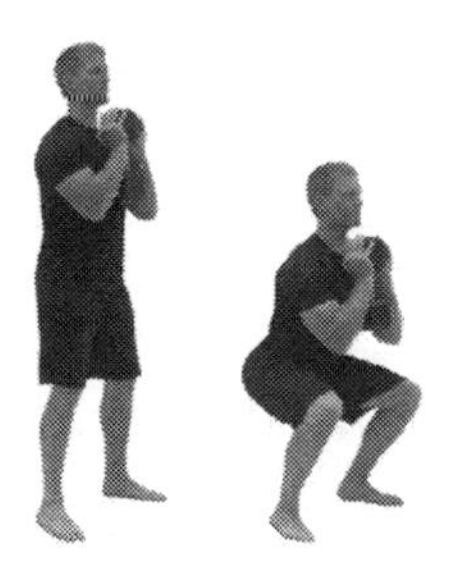

It's not only essential that we execute a variety of squatting variations to properly progress to more advanced lifts (like the Barbell Back Squat), but because training at various angles and in various positions is essential for consistent progress, maximum results, and building a strong, resilient body. For instance, a research study in 2014 in the Journal of Sports Sciences found that the 3 muscles that make up the quadriceps experienced greater activation from a Barbell Front Squat, when compared directly to the Back Squat.

Table III. Back squats and front squats mean EMG activities as a percentage of maximal voluntary isometric contraction (% MVIC), P-values, effect size (Cohen's d, Cohen, 1988) and 95% confidence intervals between descending and ascending phases, performed with 1RM loads.

	Back squat						Front squat					
	Descending phase	Ascending phase			95% CI		Descending phase	Ascending phase			95% CI	
Muscle	(mean ± s)	(mean ± s)	P	d	L	U	(mean ± s)	(mean ± s)	P	d	L	U
Rectus femoris	37.9 ± 12.1	36.0 ± 13.8	0.435	−0.15	−3.562	−7.432	46.4 ± 24.4	46.7 ± 19.4	0.932	0.01	−7.122	6.500
Vastus medialis	48.3 ± 14.5	49.3 ± 13.9	0.617	0.07	−5.293	3.286	55.1 ± 19.5	58.9 ± 17.1*	0.35*	0.32	−11.036	−.533
Vastus lateralis	45.9 ± 13.9	48.5 ± 17.2	0.225	0.17	−7.005	1.821	48.0 ± 15.8	56.2 ± 22.2	0.68	0.43	−17.190	0.7269
Erector spinae	41.1 ± 14.0	46.0 ± 17.6	0.124	0.31	−11.286	1.564	45.1 ± 12.0	48.1 ± 16.8	0.451	0.20	−11.276	5.367
Gluteus maximus	28.8 ± 18.9	47.3 ± 27.7*	0.000*	0.78	−25.816	−11.200	30.0 ± 23.0	46.5 ± 30.1*	0.000*	0.62	−22.098	−11.158
Biceps femoris	18.7 ± 14.9	34.9 ± 18.2*	0.000*	0.97	−19.740	−12.600	19.7 ± 23.3	29.5 ± 28.7*	0.001*	0.38	−14.864	−4.711
Semitendinosus	15.0 ± 6.9	29.0 ± 16.2*	0.001*	1.05	−20.720	−7.280	14.0 ± 8.1	18.4 ± 10.1*	0.036*	0.48	−8.404	−0.343

Note. * Significantly higher EMG activities during the ascending phase compared to the descending phase ($P < 0.05$).

Arguably, this is the result of a high-proportion of knee-loading, as the research noted less forward trunk lean and hamstring activation in the front squat. Meaning the quads were more active because the upright body position facilitated less hip-loading.

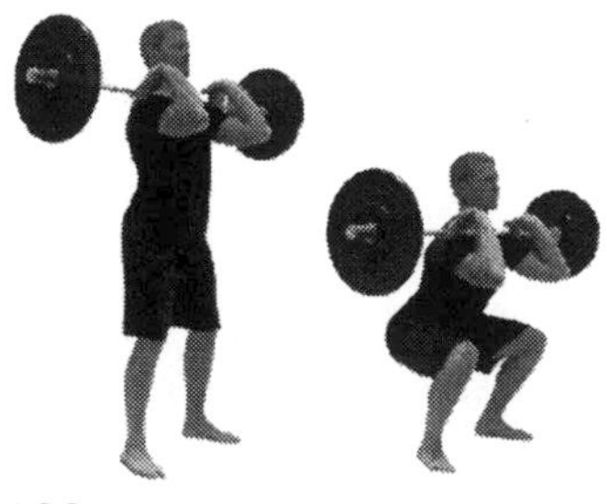

Interestingly, the quad activation during the Front Squat has also proven equivalent to the Back Squat when using lighter weights. Implying that we can achieve maximal muscle activation with squatting variations other than a Barbell Back Squat, and with a variety of loading options (heavy and light).

As you'll experience throughout *1% Fitness*, a small alteration in any of the squat movements, introduces new stressors that will challenge your body in different ways. You will like some, and you will not like others, but it's important that you work towards getting better at ALL of them.

Executing the Squat

Along with the pictures above, and the video demonstrations I've included at http://1percentworkouts.com here are some general guidelines for executing a proper squat:

1. Stand with your feet flat and slightly turned out.
2. Align your feet with your shoulders or slightly wider. *Note: Those with longer femurs (distance from knee to hip), will need to widen their base.*
3. Fix your gaze at something in front of you, position your head parallel with the ground, and bring your chest up while retracting your shoulders.
4. Distribute the weight evenly across your feet (heels down), and keep your core tight throughout the entire movement.
5. Start your descend by hinging slightly at the hips, and then bending the knees, hips, and ankles simultaneously.

6. Look to maintain an upright upper body position, by holding a tight slightly arched trunk.
7. The line of your hips should be parallel to the ground (not shifted to one side), and knees should stay in line with feet or slightly wider (not turning in).
8. Ideally, the angle of your torso should be parallel with the angle of your lower leg (tibia), and the knees should not excessively pass the toes (they will slightly).
9. For the inflexible, continue to descend until you can't go any lower without rounding your spine (butt wink). For the flexible, continue to descend until your hamstrings touch your calves (provided there's no butt wink). *Note: Anything beyond the butt wink adds too much load on the spine.*
10. When pushing up from the bottom, try to raise your shoulders and hips at the same constant speed. *Note: Picture yourself 'leading with the chest*

Squatting Depth

Aside from our Daily Deep Squat Hold (bodyweight), you need to avoid squatting to a point where you're experiencing a posterior pelvic tilt or butt wink (when the spine starts to tuck under). It's not a big deal when you do it without weight, but when there's a bar on your back or front, it places the load directly on the base of your spine.

To determine when this occurs you can try doing a lightly loaded or bodyweight squat in the mirror, or you can get on all 4's with knees spread and try to sit back. This will also give you an idea of the optimal width for your feet and knees:

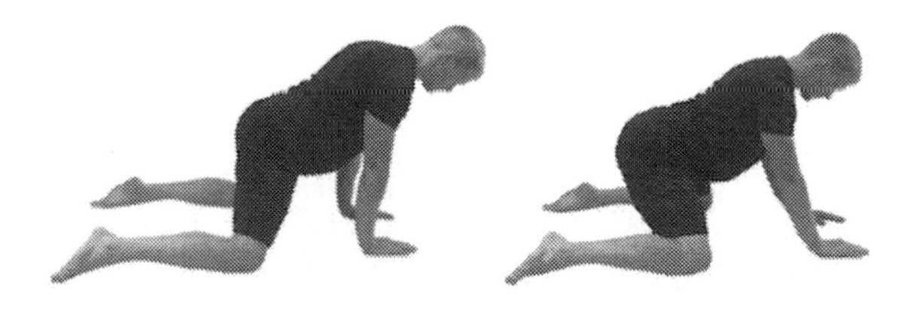

You've gone too low when your spine is no longer flat and your butt attempts to tuck underneath. Like this:

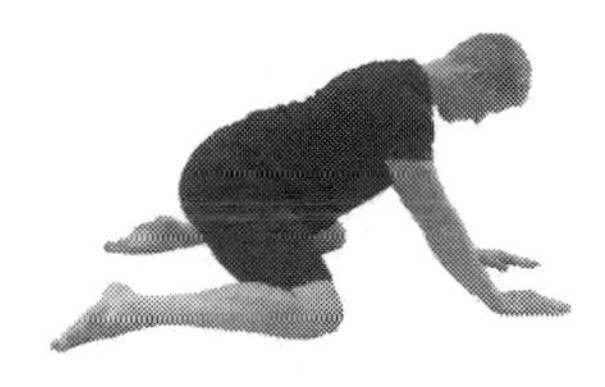

Lack of depth usually stems from poor mobility (specifically in the ankles and hips), and a weak core or glutes. Many times, it's that individuals are not engaging their core and glutes while squatting, which is why it's a good idea to practice this while the weights are light and the movements are basic.

Fortunately, your glutes and core will be getting stronger, and your overall hip and ankle mobility will improve as we progress through the various phases of *1% Fitness*. If your ankle flexibility continues to let you down, try adding in some hard dorsiflexion (opposite of toe point) stretches prior to training, or consider elevating your heels with 2.5 or 5lb plate while squatting.

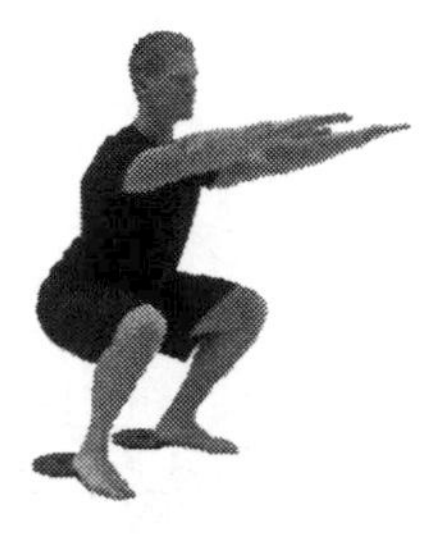

If after a few weeks, you're still not seeing depth improvements, you may just not be a deep squatter…and that's okay! Genetics come into play, and it could be anything from your femur length to your pelvic type. Take a look at the four different pelvises on the next page:

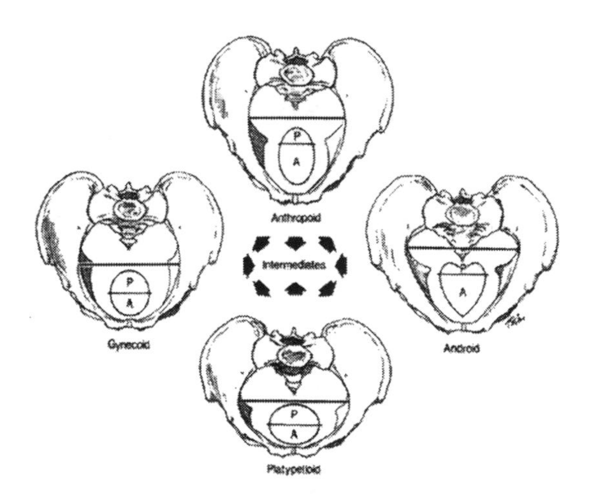

Not all are good for squatting, or as Dr. Ryan DeBell puts it:

> "There are narrow squatters and there are wide squatters. That may have nothing to do with tight muscles or "tight" joint capsules and have EVERYTHING to do with bony hip anatomy."

Locating individuals that are very good at both the squat and deadlift is rare. Generally speaking, someone with a longer torso and shorter limbs does better on the squat, while their anti-anatomical counterpart performs better in the deadlift. The short-armers can't quite get the bar off the ground in a deadlift without feeling strain in their low back and scraping their shins. And the long-leggers feel like they're going to fall on their ass if they sit back in a squat, and need to apply a lot more pressure (some suggest 30%+) to get the bar from 90 degrees to standing.

You are likely one or the other, and you'll have to get used to it. As both are essential components of developing the strong, athletic, injury-free physique we're after. Fortunately, you'll be exposed to a variety of squatting and hip hinging options, which should keep things exciting no matter your limb-torso-type. The long-leggers usually appreciate Front Squats and Goblet Squats more than Back Squats; and the short-armers usually do a lot better with Glute Bridges and Romanian Deadlifts than Barbell Bent-Knee Deadlifts.

Either way, you should aspire to get to something that's better than today in both movements. As you bend and extend more frequently and improve your strength, mobility, stability, and body awareness,

I'll bet it's somewhere lower than where you are at now. Just be sure to keep form and spine top of mind!

Major Upper Body Movements – Push & Pull

The two primary actions of the upper body – push (or press) and pull – are not only most relevant to our hunter-gatherer lineage, but they recruit the most muscle fibers.

> Research from 2010 in the Journal Strength and Conditioning Research showed significant muscle activation in 7 muscle of the back, trunk, and pecs, during a pull-up: latissimus dorsi (117-130%), biceps brachii (78-96%), infraspinatus (71-79%), lower trapezius (45-56%), pectoralis major (44-57%), erector spinae (39-41%), and external oblique (31-35%).

When compared to the lower body, the upper body is a little more straightforward; mainly because the 2 movements are the exact opposite of one another. The only difference being, where the resistance is applied. For example, take a look at the overhead push:

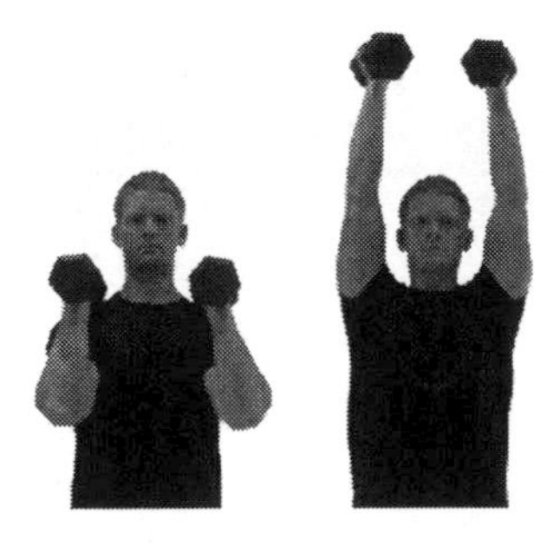

It's hard to push the arms up because of the weight of the dumbbell. While on the incline pulldown (the picture below), it's hard to pull the weight down because of the resistance from the high cable.

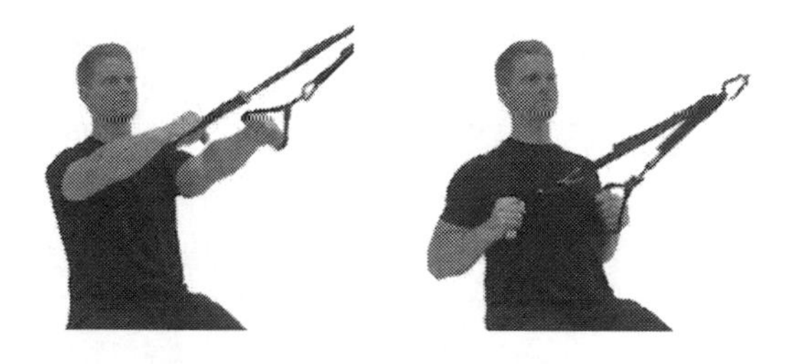

Generally speaking, the pulling movement trains the biceps, upper back, and posterior deltoid (back of shoulder), while the pushing movement trains the triceps, pectorals, and anterior deltoid (front of shoulder). And as far as training the upper body goes, this pretty much covers everything. Since even the tiny external and internal rotator muscles of the shoulder are training during pressing and pulling movements (...especially with the various angles and grip positions you'll experience with *1% Fitness*).

For both the push and pull, we're after a full range of motion at each end of the movement. Meaning full stretch of the pecs and shoulders or lats and biceps after the eccentric portion, and full tricep lockout or upper back contraction after the forceful push or pull.

Despite the commonly cited misconception that 'bringing a barbell to your chest is bad for your shoulders,' the opposite is in fact true. Like we discussed earlier, you get injured from not training your muscles to full range; as unfortunately, life and sport don't stop at 90 degrees. Full-range of motion is how you achieve fully developed and fully functional muscles that are flexible, attractive, and injury-free.

Proper Form – Scaps & Bows

For most pressing exercises, the elbows won't be completely tight to the body, but maintaining at least a 45-degree angle between your upper arm and core is ideal. Especially if you're new to weight training and learning these movements for the first time.

If you're new to weight training, it's especially critical that you perfect a healthy elbow position from the outset. The introductory bodyweight phase (Phase 1) is the ideal time to work on perfecting a healthy elbow position, as we typically see them flaring on the push-up. To ensure proper execution, you'll want to keep your incline push-up as high as is necessary before progressing to a lower elevation.

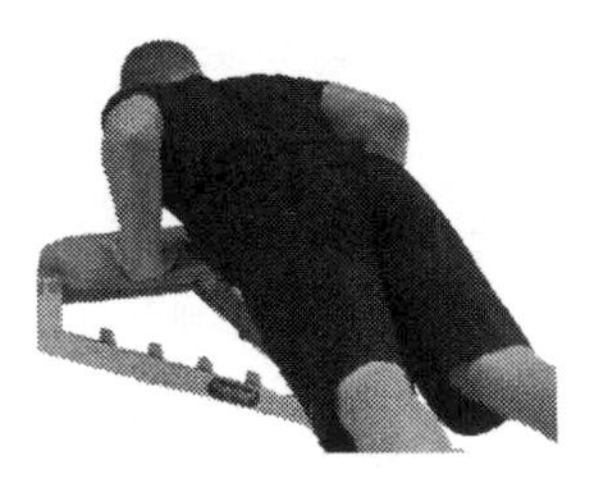

While we're on the topic, maintaining a tight (or stable) core throughout this movement is also a requirement before progressing. For both the push-up, and the plank, the torso needs to be somewhere between arching the back and sticking the butt out. And since over-arching tends to be more common, chances are you'll need to practice flexing your butt and trying to tuck it under (like the camel).

> Fun Fact: Each push-up variation lifts a different percent of your bodyweight – 41% with hands elevated on a 24-inch bench (less from higher up), 49% with hands on the floor and from knees, 64% with hands on the floor and from feet (standard pushup), and 75% with hands on floor and feet on a 24-inch bench (more from higher up).

During overhead pressing the elbows aren't necessarily at a 45-degree angle, as much as they're in front where you can see them. That being said, there still needs to be a conscious effort to keep them 'in' (or 'forward') during the lowering and pressing of the bar.

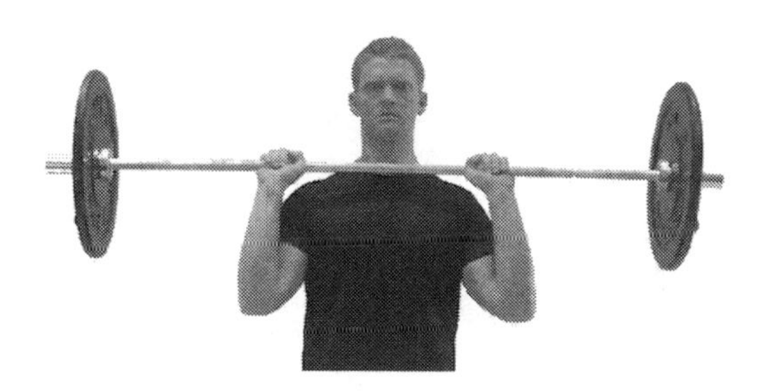

Over-focusing on the elbows during the slower eccentric portion is a great way to teach yourself and your shoulders the correct movement pattern.

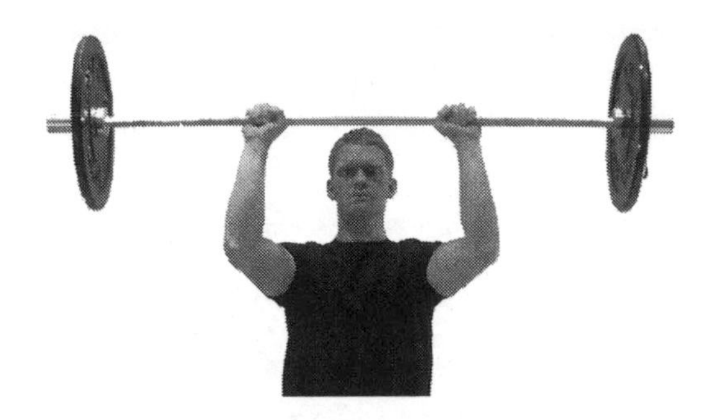

The elbows will no doubt flare slightly on the push, but it should be minimal, and the intent to keep them 'in' should always be present.

"Concentration on the way down. Intention on the way up."

This same intent needs to be applied to the retraction of the shoulder during pulling movements. Which as we discussed in Principle #1, involves drawing your shoulders down and back, and trying to pull the points of your shoulder blades together.

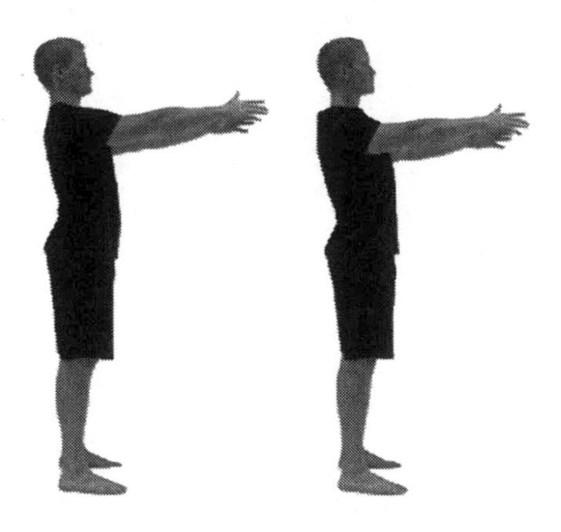

Like most things, the best way to perfect it, is to practice it. If you're unsatisfied with your ability to 'retract your scaps,' look to add one or several of the useful progressions below into your dynamic warm-up or daily routine. In all cases, the arms remain locked-out completely, the body stays still, and the shoulders slide back and forth.

The Push Away – Back Against Wall or Back on Floor

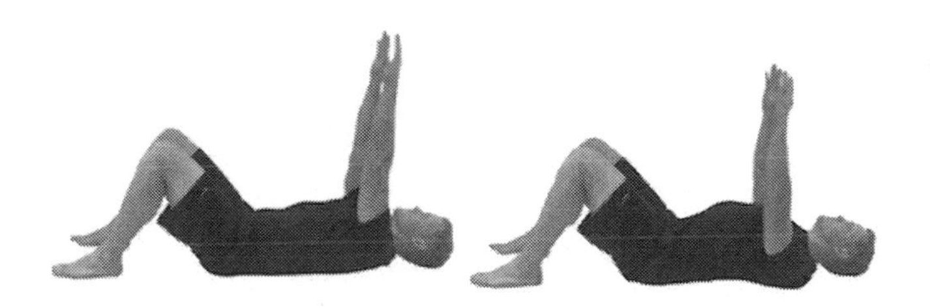

The Push Off – From Wall, Bench, or Floor

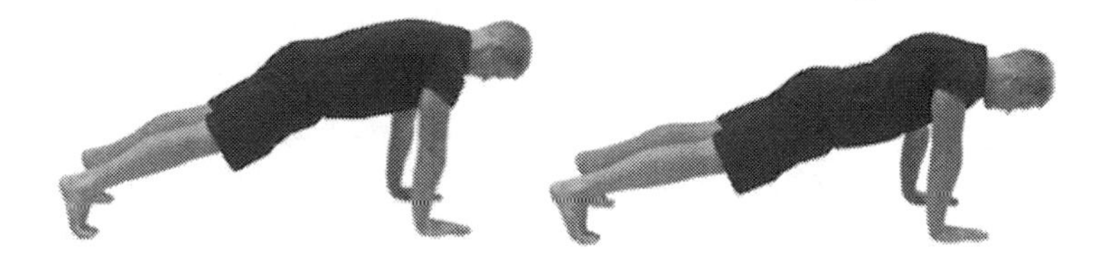

The Pull Down – From High-Pulley or Chin-Up Bar

Executing the scapular retraction correctly is key to developing a bigger back, and healthy shoulders. Those new to resistance training need to take the time to learn and perfect this movement, and those experienced in training need to be sure they've got it down pat. Your pulls, posture, and performance will thank you!

Unilateral (1-Arm or 1-Leg) Exercises

Both unilateral (1 limb) and bilateral (2 limbs) exercises are encouraged for the upper and lower body, as performing 1-leg or 1-arm movements improves the strength in 2-leg or 2-arm movements, and visa versa.

In some instances, a unilateral movement tends to work better and feel more natural because it permits better range of motion. 1-leg or 1-arm can also supply greater core activation and muscle activation compared to their 2-leg or 2-arm equivalent. For example, some top Strength Coaches have argued that a single-leg exercise like the Back Foot Elevated (Bulgarian) Lunge is more effective at loading the quads than a Barbell Back Squat.

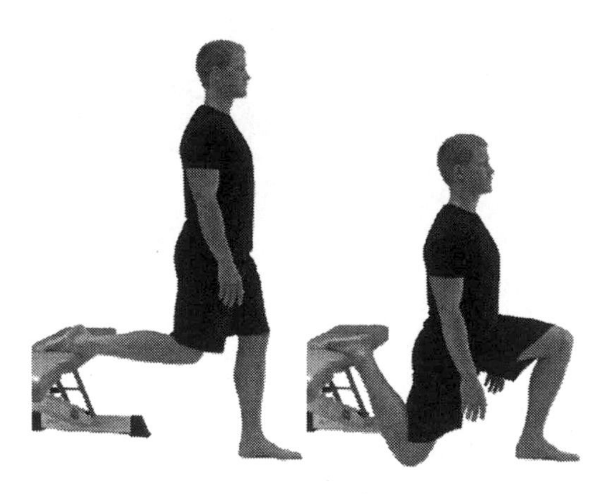

And it's not hard to see how one could make a similar case for the 1-Arm Dumbbell Row and the Back.

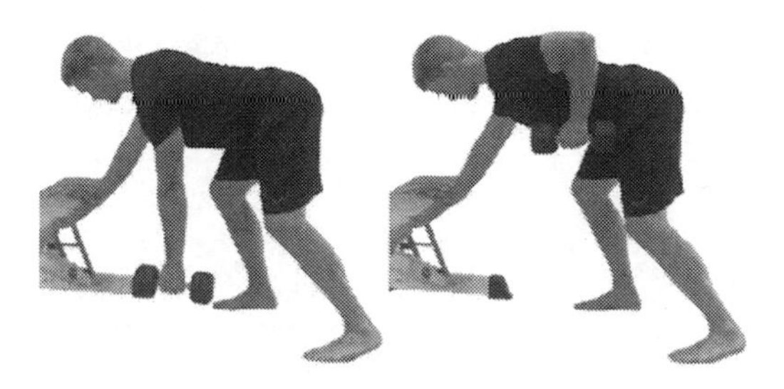

Interestingly, a research study from 2012 in the Journal of Strength and Conditioning Research determined that the Back Foot Elevated Lunge had a slightly higher testosterone response than the traditional bilateral Back Squat.

That being said, unilateral exercises are less efficient, which is why I suggest limiting yourself to 1 per workout (upper or lower). You should also look to reserve them for superset #2 (the B's), as performing the big bilateral compound movements to late in the workout can hamper performance.

> "It is recommended that strength programs sequence exercises to optimize the preservation of exercise intensity (large before small muscle group exercises, multiple-joint exercises before single-joint exercises, and higher-intensity before lower-intensity exercises)."
> *American College of Sports Medicine*

Complimentary Core Movements – Twist & Resist

When most people think of core training, they immediately think of crunches and sit-ups. Because bending forward to get your back off the ground and crunch your abs with a flexed spine is the best way to get a 6-pack right?

As your learned in *Live It NOT Diet!,* abs are made in the kitchen, not the weight room. And as far as building a great core goes, the best way to make your abs pop is to perform free-weight compound exercises.

Despite the conventional prescription of doing thousands of crunches per day, the abdominal fibers respond best when fighting to stabilize heavy weights.

> Research from the Journal of Strength & Conditioning Research in 2013 found that the abdominal muscles were better activated with integrated core exercises (glutes and shoulders recruited at the same time), as opposed to complete isolation.

Some have described the core as a box with the abs at the front, glutes and paraspinals in the back, hip girdle and pelvic floor at the bottom, and diaphragm at the top. And others have referred to it as the anatomy between the knees and the sternum, with an emphasis on the abdominals, low back, and hips. But either way, it encompasses a lot more that those 6-8 little guys some of us can see in the front.

> When we speak of the core we mean the whole musculature of the torso – glutes, low back (erectors), hip flexors, obliques, etc.

This is the reason free-weight compound exercises (pushing, pulling, bending, and extending) are best for the core; as all the muscles are firing to stabilize our body. Think of the squat for example, where the core is preventing the spine and pelvis from flexing and extending from front to back and side-to-side (laterally), while making sure the hips are not adducting/abducting or internally/externally rotating in any one direction.

But that being said, we can further develop our resistance to these multi-directional movements (stability), and gain higher levels of strength and performance, by performing core work that's aligned with our laborious past. Basically, these exercises will be performed at the END of your *1% Fitness* workouts (to avoid pre-fatiguing the core and harming performance), and for simplicity they're classified into 2 categories:

Resist - is the core's primary responsibility. It's often performed subconsciously, as a small degree of resistance takes place when our body fights to keep us upright and avoid forward, backward, and sideways bending (i.e. flexion or extension). From a hunter-gatherers perspective, core training was common during carrying, which we will experiment with in Phase 2.

Twist - is the other major action of the core. It's usually involved in throwing actions, or when picking something up or down on an angle. Although it's commonly tackled by inexperienced trainees, it's definitely an advanced core movement. Don't expect to see any twisting movements until the more advanced workouts in Phase 3.

Similar to the other 4 movements, the core will be isolated to the point where you feel the muscles being worked, but we'll be training it on a more functional platform.

The Primary Core Movement – Resist

One of the greatest resistance exercises to develop a solid core is the plank. And based on the amount of repetitions we'll be doing that resist flexion of the spine (deadlift, squats, etc.) it provides a healthy balance of extension resistance. Here is the proper way to perform a plank, and 4 critical coaching points below:

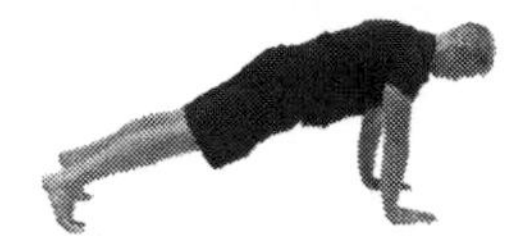

1. Position your shoulders directly over your hands.
2. Squeeze your glutes and slightly round your spine to prevent extension (avoid arching).
3. Pull your feet and hands into the ground as if you're trying to bring them towards each other (the ground will prevent that).
4. When you're no longer fully activated with your glutes and hands & feet, the plank is finished. Remember, we're looking for quality (intensity) not quantity (duration).

Aside from your standard front and side planks, there are a tremendous number of challenging dynamic plank exercises that are classified as 'Active Planks.' Expect to perform a few of them in Phase 1, and during the High-Intensity Interval Training (HIIT) workouts in Phase 3.

Isometric Holds and Weighted Carries (or Farmers Walks) are the primary 'Resist' exercise that are a requirement in addition to your standard push-pull multi-joint movements. Along with giving you the opportunity to work on your posture and increase your daily step count, they can improve your core resistance in 4 different directions – anti-flexion, anti-extension, anti-lateral flexion (left & right).

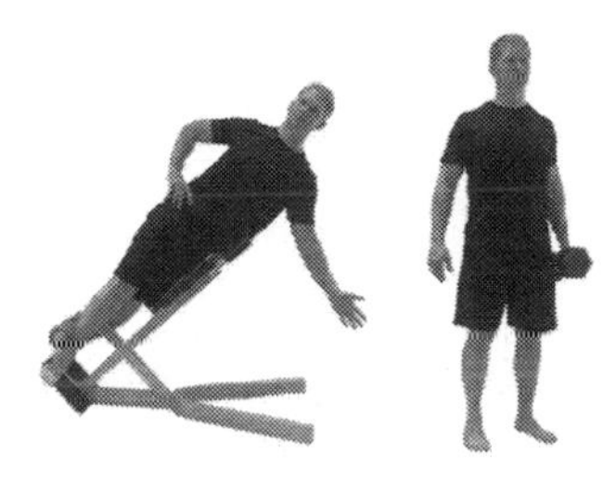

We will also be looking to prevent rotation (twisting). But for beginners especially, the best anti-rotation exercise is the Paloff Press. Generally it's performed with a pulley, but it's possible to accomplish the same result in a variety of different ways (ex: resistance band).

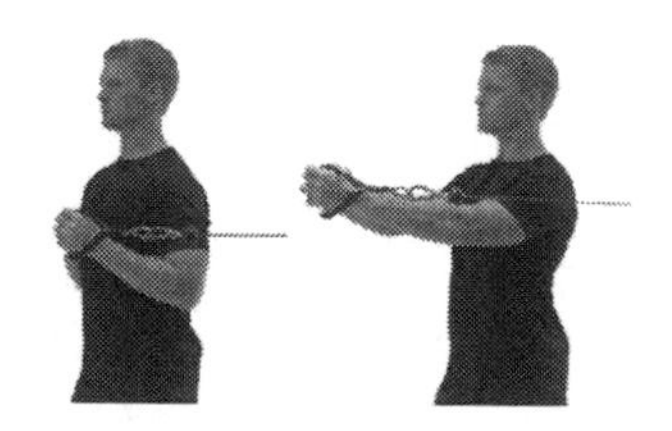

All of these exercises form the building blocks of a strong core that's ready to upgrade to the more challenging twisting moves in the later phases of *1% Fitness*.

The Secondary Core Movement – Twist

Twist (or rotation) not only encompasses a toss or throw from one side of the body to the other, but it includes the bending, thrusting, and off-center movement patterns that were necessary for the hunter-gatherer to survive. Similar to the Active Planks, you'll see the dynamic version of these twisting exercises incorporated throughout the HIIT workouts in Phase 3.

> Research in the Strength and Conditioning Journal in 2011 highlights evidence suggesting that dynamic core movements are superior to isometric core movements for muscle hypertrophy.

That being said, learning to activate and fire the muscles needed to stabilize the core in a variety of positions is essential before attempting any weight-training movements and more dynamic core exercises. Not to scare you, but research suggests that progressing too quickly to dynamic spinal exercises can negatively affect the discs. Likewise, performing these all-encompassing core movements improperly (excessive end-ranges, etc.) can produce a similar outcome. The exercises are definitely safe, but it's essential that you develop a solid base that gives you the ability to properly control your core in all directions. This is why the body-weight exercises in Phase 1 place a considerable focus on exercises that promote activation of the glutes, lower back, and abdominals.

Interestingly, research from back specialist, Dr. Stu McGill suggests that muscular endurance of the core is more important than muscular strength for preventing low back pain and injury. Meaning, body-weight core exercises for high-reps are well worth your time and attention. By checking your ego at the door, and being patient with Phase 1, you'll 'Restore Your Core' and quickly be on your way to a bulletproof midsection.

"For 90 percent of people, 90 percent of the time, total-body training is the way to go."

— Tony Gentilcore

Superset Upper With Lower & Push With Pull

Although personal trainers, strength coaches, and exercise specialists across the globe may use the term in different ways, they'd all agree that supersetting is the most efficient way to train. Heck, they'd probably have trouble disagreeing with me saying it's also the most effective way to train.

> In 1% Fitness, the term 'superset' means alternating between two exercises with non-competing muscle groups, instead of doing all sets of 1 exercise before moving onto the next.

Basically, supersetting gets you to perform a second exercise in the time that would've been wasted standing around waiting to recover from the first. For example, you could do 10 reps of Incline Dumbbell Bench Press and rest for 90 seconds before doing another set, or you could do 10 reps of Incline Dumbbell Bench Press, follow it up with 10 reps of Back Extensions, and rest for 60 seconds. Instead of twiddling your thumbs for 90 seconds, you spent 30 of those 90 seconds doing another exercise that used different (non-competing) muscle groups.

Example:

A1 – Incline Dumbbell Bench Press - 4sets - 10reps - 0sec rest

A2 – 45 Degree Back Extension - 4sets - 10reps - 60sec rest

.Perform a set of Bench Press, go immediately to Back Extension (0sec rest), and then rest for 60sec.

.When the 60sec rest is up, do another set of Bench Press, move immediately to Back Extension, and take another 60sec rest

.Repeat that routine (the A's) until you've completed 4 sets of each; then move on to the next superset (the B's)

Aside from creating shorter workouts, and freeing up extra time in your life, supersetting leads to better results.

Supersetting - Higher Testosterone

Since we're here to build muscle and not burn it, our workout efficiency is extremely important. Supersetting keeps your total workout time short, so you can take advantage of higher levels of testosterone and lower levels of cortisol. As we discussed in *Eat Meat And Stop Jogging*, a high Testosterone-to-Cortisol (T:C) ratio promotes muscle building (anabolism), while a low T:C ratio favors muscle loss (catabolism).

> Testosterone peaks and starts to fall after 20-30 minutes, while cortisol continues to rise throughout a workout session.

Supersetting not only produces a more favorable hormonal environment that builds muscle, but it gives us the ability to perform a high volume when these hormones are at their highest. The more work, or volume we can get in earlier, the more successful we will be in our lifts and the better our adaptive response will be in the form of strength and muscle development.

For example, if you completed 6 exercises in a workout with 4 sets of each exercise, you'd complete a total of 24 sets. Without supersetting, this workout would take at least 48 minutes (24 sets with 30 seconds work & 90 seconds rest). With supersetting, it would only take 24 minutes (12 supersets with 60 seconds work & 60 seconds rest), to perform the same total volume with equivalent recovery (90 seconds after each exercise).

In the supersetting option, all sets and reps are performed while testosterone levels are at their highest; and arguably, when energy levels are at their highest. In both cases, this translates to an increased probability of lifting heavier weights and completing more reps; which equates to better strength and muscle development.

> "Multiple set resistance-training protocols of moderate to high intensity, using short rest intervals and stressing a large muscle mass may be optimal as they appear to produce the greatest acute hormonal elevations" Sports Medicine, 2005

The secretions of muscle building hormones (GH, testosterone) are far greater following high-volume training with short rest-periods, compared to low-volume training with long rest-periods. Aside from building a stronger well-muscled physique, these elevations in hormones and exercise by-products result in significantly greater fat loss, and post-exercise caloric burn (EPOC).

Supersetting - Higher Metabolic Stress

Supersets also lead to better results because of something called metabolic stress. Along with mechanical tension, muscle damage, and hormonal processes (IGF-1, Testosterone, GH), metabolic stress has been identified as one of the main drivers of muscle growth (hypertrophy). With many researchers suggesting it may be the most critical.

Generally, it's referred to as the 'pump,' and it's based on the amount of excess stress and exercise by-products (blood, lactate, etc.) in the muscles. Although the easiest way to achieve this is to consistently overwork the muscle by shortening the rest period and repping-out to failure, this isn't the best approach.

Why?

Because the muscles being trained become overly fatigued, and we end up lifting lighter weights for a lot less reps. This not only decreases the mechanical tension and volume, but it pushes us into the muscular endurance zone as the time under tension (TUT) is far too high and rest period far too short.

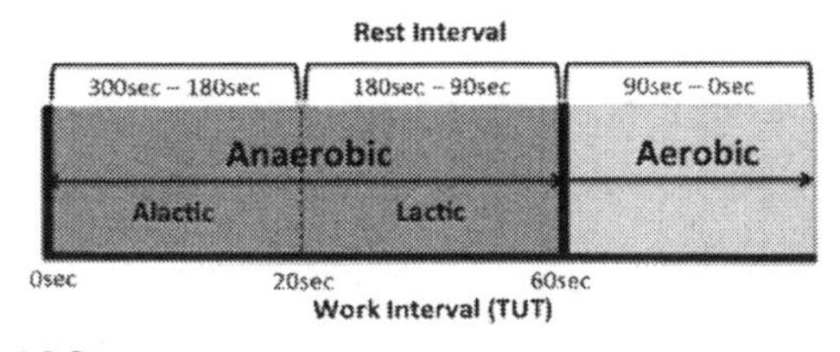

When our training becomes 'aerobic,' instead of 'anaerobic,' we experience a negative shift in fiber type (Type II to Type I), and we fail to build the strength and muscle we started lifting weights for in the first place.

The best way to maximize the pump without minimizing strength is to stay in the proper work-to-rest ratio. And aside from the optimal training variables we'll discuss in Principle #6, we accomplish this by supersetting. For instance, performing a movement like the squat with a row or pulldown adds additional stress to that movement. Although, unlike shortening rest or repping to failure, it doesn't prefatigue the muscles. We experience the hypertrophic benefits from an increase in metabolic stress and muscle-building hormones, while maximizing the strength potential of the exercise.

In many cases, that strength potential is greater. Arguably, because of the increase in circulating hormones. For example, research from 2009 in the Journal of Sports Sciences compared a group performing traditional single-exercise training on the bench press, with a group supersetting the bench press with a pulling movement. After 8 weeks, the superset group had greater strength gains on the bench press.

Another study from 2005 in the Journal of Strength and Conditioning research tested rugby players with a significant amount of training experience, and found that those supersetting a pulling movement with a bench press throw had a 4.7% greater increase in power than those performing the bench press throw on it's own.

Whether this means strength and power gains are better with supersetting is debatable, but clearly they're not harmed. You can perform the same amount of work, and make similar gains with half the time commitment.

Supersetting – In Our Genes

The superior hormonal environment, elevated performance potential, increased metabolic stress, and ability to do the same workload in half the time should provide enough support to superset in the first place. However, we can also take a look at the movement regimen of our hunter-gatherer ancestors, and justify supersetting based on that. As aside from performing multi-joint movements instead of single-joint, overcoming resistance at various angles, and strengthening the body as one unit, there was no methodical approach to their physical labor.

The hunter-gatherers likely did a combination of upper and lower body movements at one time, and various muscle groups were stressed (including those of the core). They weren't only climbing trees on Monday's, and only picking up rocks on Thursdays. They were likely doing both on the same day, and more than likely doing both movements at once.

Now, don't get me wrong. I'm not saying we have to exercise just like a hunter-gatherer, as clearly weight-training in a commercial gym facility is far from primal. Although, it's worth considering when trying to determine the optimal exercise roadmap that's most closely related to our genetics.

Plus, it's an appropriate mindset to have while reading the next recommendation.

Superset Upper & Lower Body Movements

Staying on the topic of ancestral movement, I think it's reasonable to think that the hunter-gatherer never skipped leg day. In fact, when looking at the various movements that were probably performed on a regular basis it's hard to find one that doesn't involve the legs. As we often lunge down to aid a throw, and squat or jump to initiate climbing.

> "The transition to agriculture in Central Europe, reduced the need for long-distance travel or heavy physical work....fewer people were regularly doing tasks that were very strenuous on their legs."
> –Alison Macintosh, Anthropologist

That being said, the scientific reason for training upper and lower body together is because the legs excite the nervous system more than the upper body. Squats, deadlifts, and lunges really get the heart pumping, and hormones flowing, and this ends up getting utilized at whatever exercise we decide to superset it with.

> Research from 2011 in the Journal of Applied Physiology compared an upper-lower superset routine with an upper-only routine, and found far greater increases in testosterone and growth hormone, and arm strength and power in the upper-lower superset group.

By taking that fired up energy from an all-encompassing leg exercise over to an upper-body movement - like the bench press - we expose the pecs and shoulders to higher hormonal concentrations in the blood, and this leads to more push. Meaning, heavier weights for more reps and superior strength and muscle development.

> In an 11-week study in the Journal of Strength and Conditioning Research from 2010, a group assigned to an upper-lower superset saw significant hormonal increases, and far greater strength, muscle, and power gains, compared to an upper-only group that saw none (while performing the same total volume).

The crazy part is, the gains from upper-lower workouts are even greater with less training. For instance, research from 1994 in the Canadian Journal of Applied Physiology divided 30 young women into 2 groups:

- Upper-lower combined training 2 times per week
- Upper-lower split training 4 times per week

Despite only completing half the training sessions, the whole body group had better increases in muscle mass for the trunk (3.4 vs. 2.7%) and legs (4.9% vs. 1.7%), and total muscle mass overall (4.1 vs. 2.6%).

A study from 2011 in the Journal of Strength and Conditioning Research came to the same conclusion when comparing total-body training (upper & lower) 3 times per week with upper-lower split training 4 times per week (2 upper, 2 lower). Even though both groups performed 72 sets per week for 8-12 repetitions with weights corresponding to 50-80% of their 1 rep max, the researchers found greater increases in muscle mass with the total body routine (3.1% vs. 1.5%).

Whether this is the result of an elevated hormonal surge from the lower body movements, or simply because it targets the same muscle groups numerous times per week, this is clearly something we should be practicing. Especially if we're seeking bigger gains with a smaller time commitment.

The practical reason for training upper and lower body together is because training legs on their own SUCKS. Experience has taught me that the motivation for workouts where you're training 'only legs' is extremely low, and there's a much higher likelihood that you'll skip your workout or put forth a half ass effort. By keeping legs and upper body together we operate in a work-for-reward system, similar to the one presented in *Live It NOT Diet!* Eat good for 6 days of the week, and enjoy whatever you want for 1. Go for a 30-min walk in the morning, and enjoy some fruit with your breakfast. Fire off 10 reps of Dumbbell Deadlifts, and enjoy 10 reps of Flat Barbell Bench Press.

This is the system I use with my clients, and the same strategy I follow myself. It works because every workout is upper body, and this means you won't miss your workouts. More importantly, you won't miss legs, and leg exercises are critical for developing the strong, attractive, balanced physique we're striving for.

Superset Push & Pull Movements

Even though we're supersetting muscle groups on opposite ends of the body, there's more competing variables than you might think; and this can hurt our execution. Despite a few pairings that are just too hard, the 2 biggest considerations in executing a non-conflicting upper-lower superset are grip and core. Thus, as you can see from the grouping below, we avoid putting Upper Body Pull with Lower Body Pull, because of grip fatigue:

- Upper Body Push –Lower Body Pull (Extend)
- Upper Body Pull – Lower Body Push (Bend)

This also works well because Upper Body Push and Lower Body Push (Bend) seem to be a little too physically taxing. With Squat and Bench Press being the perfect example.

If the rule confuses you, here's an alternative way of thinking about it:

- Pull & Bend
- Push & Extend

Unfortunately, there is the potential for 'core' conflicts, but the workouts in *1% Fitness* have been carefully designed and tested with this in mind. As you excel through the various phases, and get a better feel for which muscles are fatiguing, you'll start to understand the best exercise combinations. And for those that don't, there's an option discussed at the end of the book regarding ongoing program support.

Based on our 'Upper with Lower' and 'Push with Pull' groupings, here are the 4 possible ways you can structure your workout:

A1) Push - A2) Extend
B1) Pull – B2) Bend

A1) Pull – A2) Bend
B1) Push – B2) Bend

A1) Extend – A2) Push
B1) Bend; B2) Pull

A2) Bend – A2) Pull
B1) Extend; B2) Push

Notice that the position of the exercises in the workout doesn't change what movement they're supersetted or grouped with. We always keep Pulls with Bends and Pushes with Extends.

Since I believe in earning your upper body lifts, expect to see the workouts looking more like the 2nd two options (i.e. legs first!) Plus, more reps are achieved in the exercises performed first, so it makes sense to start with the big bilateral leg movements (i.e. squat or dead!)

You'll notice the motivation to push the limits with your legs is less appealing than the upper body, and this desire continues to decline as the workout progresses. No one minds forcing upper body presses to get the shoulders and chest a little more pumped up, but the desire to do the same with the legs once fatigue sets in and hormone levels diminish is not ideal.

When you make it to the end of this book, and start looking at the workouts, you'll notice we always start with either a Squat (Bend) or Deadlift (Extend). Phase 2 is our opportunity to get familiar with these movements, until we transition to more advanced barbell and unilateral progressions at the end of Phase 3.

"High Load Training increases muscle mass. Low Load Training increases muscle mass. Moral of story, lift weights consistently."

— Jeremy Loenneke

PRINCIPLE #6

Alternate Between Strength & Muscle Building

"How many reps should I be doing to gain muscle?"

"I lift weights 2 times a week; is that enough?

"My friend told me I need at least 2 minutes of rest when training for strength…?"

"How many sets should I be doing for each body part?"

Not to worry, these questions make my head spin too. The reality is, resistance training can be damn confusing…if you let it!

Fortunately for you, I've taken the necessary time to find answers to all of these questions; and I've organized all the information into an easy-to-follow chart.

Program Design – Keep it Simple Stupid

When designing a program the first question to answer is 'what is the training goal?' Since I know it's a better body and a longer stronger life, I'll answer that for you:

Strength & Muscle

In order to develop strength and muscle in the free-weight compound exercises we already reviewed, we need to select the proper reps, sets, rest, and tempo. These training variables are characteristic of all resistance training routines, and they're also where people tend to get the most confused.

The reason there's confusion is because sometimes strength gurus like to be different. And with only so many options to play with in order to set themselves apart, you can see why manipulating bar speeds, rep ranges, and set schemes becomes popular. Don't get me wrong, I love experimenting with pauses, drop sets, 1 & 1/4 reps, and bands and chains too, but for the majority of the population this is unnecessary.

My apologies for waiting until halfway through the book to tell you this, but the resistance training most should be doing is pretty straightforward. Or at least, I've done my best to comb through the research and deliver it that way.

Strength Workouts vs. Muscle Workouts

Throughout *1% Fitness*, you only need to be concerned with two types of workouts:

1. Strength Building Workouts
2. Muscle Building Workouts

Because of the way we're grouping upper & lower body and push & pull exercises together, the only difference between the workouts is going to be the training variables. Fortunately, we already know the actions involved (push, pull, bend, extend, twist/resist), and muscle groups getting trained, and this chart takes care of the rest –volume (reps and sets), intensity (rest), and movement speed (tempo).

	Set Range	Rep Range	Tempo	Total Rest
Strength	3 - 4	4 - 8	3010	2min or 60/60
Muscle	3 - 4	8 - 12	4010	1min or 30/30

These variables are determined by something called Time Under Tension (TUT), which is the amount of time the muscles being trained are under stress. And as you can see from the chart below, the total TUT varies based on the training goal of the individual:

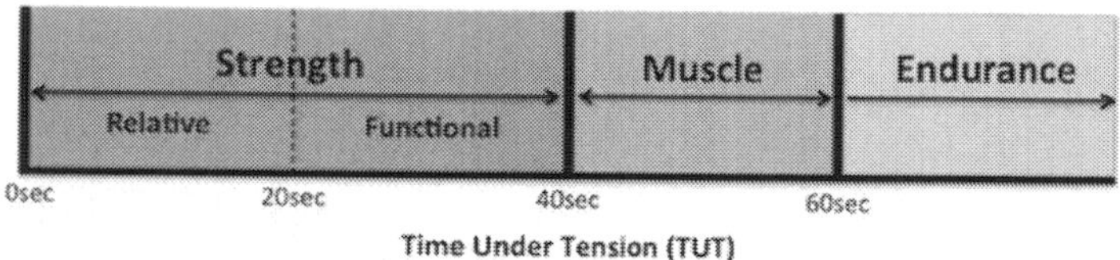

Since we're looking to build strength and muscle, we're going to stay below 60 seconds under tension. And since it's possible to build strength without lifting too heavy, we'll stay above 20 seconds the majority of the time.

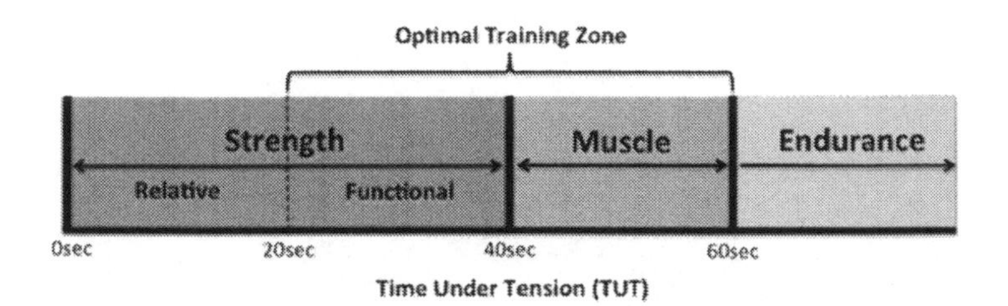

During low-rep strength workouts (4reps) we'll play on the cusp of 20 seconds, but there's no reason to risk injury seeking 1-3 rep maxes.

In general, our 'muscle workouts' put us between 40 and 60 seconds under tension, and our strength workouts put us between 20 and 40 seconds. Which as displayed in the chart from earlier, requires the right combination of repetitions (reps) and movement speed (tempo).

	Set Range	Rep Range	Tempo	Total Rest
Strength	3 - 4	4 - 8	3010	2min or 60/60
Muscle	3 - 4	8 - 12	4010	1min or 30/30

10 reps at a tempo of 4010 would equate to approximately 50 seconds under tension [10 x (4+0+1+0), and this gets us to the proper TUT for hypertrophy (muscle growth).

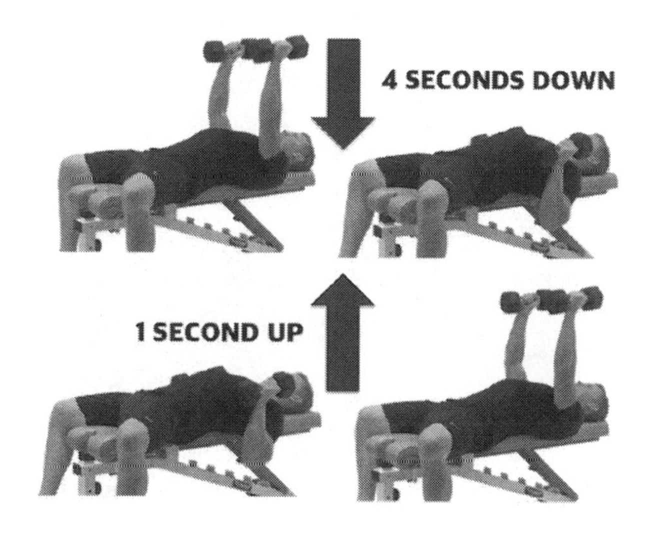

8 reps at a tempo of 3010 would be more of a strength set, as it puts us at a TUT of 32 seconds [8 x (3+0+1+0)].

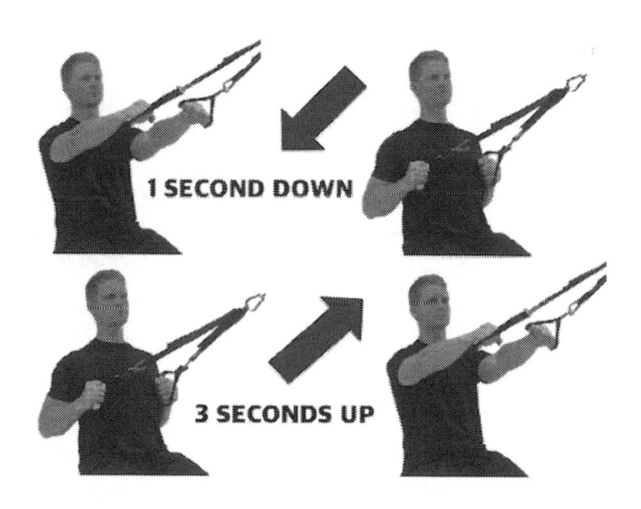

When the reps are performed with the proper tempo, we end up with the following TUT range for each type of workout:

Strength: 16sec – 32sec

Muscle: 40sec – 60sec

Putting us in the optimal rep range for strength and muscle development.

Optimal Rep Range

Research can be somewhat inconsistent in determining the optimal rep range, but it's consistently shown that performing sets of less than 15 reps is superior to sets of more than 15 reps. It's also been clear in showing that it's possible to build both muscle and strength between 4 and 12 reps per set.

Sure, strength development is greater on lower rep schemes (ex: 3-5) compared to higher ones (ex: 9-11) but research has determined that it's still possible to build strength during 'muscle building' workouts (8-12 rep range).

> "For loading (strength), it is recommended that loads corresponding to 1-12RM be used in periodized fashion with emphasis on the 6-12RM zone using 1-2min rest periods between sets at a moderate velocity." American College of Sports Medicine, 2009

This is one of the reason's we don't bother maxing out at very low (1-3) rep ranges. There's a lot less risk executing multiple reps with weight you can handle than aiming for a 1-rep max you've never attempted before. And fortunately, research points to considerable increases in maximal dynamic strength in the 4-8 rep range.

Likewise, there's substantial evidence that training relatively close to failure with moderate-to-heavy loads is superior for building strength and muscle in both trained and untrained individuals. Meaning a consistent increase in weight to a point where it's challenging in the rep range provided, will be necessary with the *1% Fitness* workouts. Not necessarily maxing-out on every set (and this isn't recommended), but having to put extra force into the last 1-2 reps in the given range.

For example, the 12th rep in a 10-12 rep range should be challenging, and if it's not, you should raise the weight. Provided of course, that the form and tempo are on-point.

The same principle applies to the 10 in the 10-12 rep range, but in reverse. If you can't complete rep 10, you should decrease the weight.

It makes sense that greater hypertrophy could be gained by reaching failure, as more muscles are recruited during fatigue to complete the given number of repetitions, and metabolic stress is elevated. Although, research also suggests that repetition failure is not critical to elicit significant neural and structural changes to skeletal muscle and consistently hitting failure could actually be detrimental.

> A study from 2006 in the Journal of Applied Physiology had participants train to failure for 16 weeks, and found considerable reductions in resting IGF-1 and testosterone suppression.

Going to full failure should be reserved for the final set on a given exercise as you don't want to be too gassed after set 1 or 2 of a 4-set superset.

Optimal Tempo

The tempos and rep ranges in the *1% Fitness* chart are the ideal mix of simple and effective. For instance, the first number in the tempo (the eccentric action) is more critical to gaining strength and muscle, and leads to far greater development than the concentric action (third number), so we spend more time there.

Tempo = 4 – 0 – 1 – 0

- Eccentric = 4 seconds
- Concentric = 1 second

A research study from 2006 in the journal Medicine and Science in Sports and Exercise, split participants into 2 groups with one doing only the eccentric part of an elbow flexion exercise and the other doing only the concentric portion. Not only was muscle development significantly higher in the eccentric group (11% vs. 3%), but they had equal improvements in concentric strength (14% vs. 18%), and far greater improvements in eccentric strength (26% vs. 9%).

Likewise, in the year 2000, researchers in the Journal Physiology tested quadriceps development and found far greater increases in strength and hypertrophy for those performing the eccentric-only training, compared to those doing concentric-only.

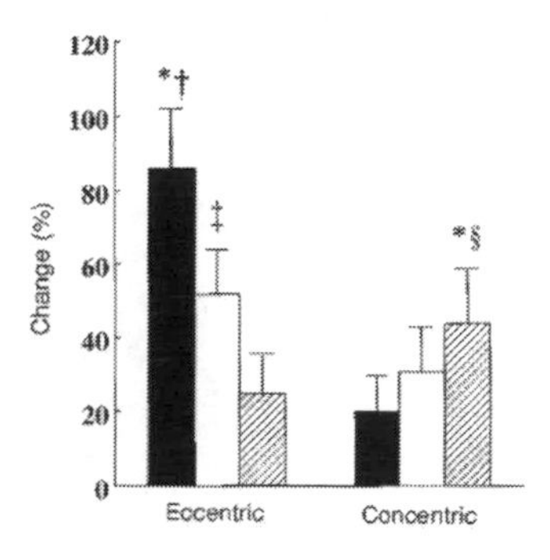

Why?

It appears the eccentric action in an exercise is less metabolically demanding (less motor unit activation required), but produces more force production per unit of muscle size. Meaning, heavier weight can be applied with less muscular stress. Or as researchers in a meta-analysis from 2009 in the British Journal of Sports Medicine put it:

> "The superiority of eccentric training to increase muscle strength and mass appears to be related to the higher loads developed during eccentric contractions."

Most of us can attest to this, as it always seems significantly easier to resist a heavy weight, than it is to push or lift one. For example, when lying on your back it's difficult to push someone off of you, and a lot easier to prevent them from getting too close.

Either way, it's clear that if we're going to focus on controlling one part of the movement to extend the TUT, we're better off spending more time in the eccentric portion. As aside from the superior force-to-stress relationship, we see greater elevations in muscle protein synthesis, superior hormonal increases (IGF-1, gH) and greater muscle tension, damage, and recruitment. Which are all factors that contribute to hypertrophic adaptation.

Lucky for us, performing the concentric action with a quicker speed (explosively) is also optimal for developing strength and muscle. Meaning, our slow eccentric and fast concentric tempos of 4010 and 3010 put us in the optimal zone for growth.

Realistically, the 1 could be swapped for an 'X,' as we usually want to execute our push or pull with explosiveness. Heavier weights will no doubt travel slower and light weights faster, but the force you apply to the bar should always be 100% if you expect to make improvements in strength.

This is also important when looking at health and longevity, as an explosive concentric concentric action increases the Type II muscle fibers that drastically decline with age.

> Humans can lose up to 40% of their muscle mass by the age of 80, with preferential reduction in the cross-sectional area (CSA) of the fast, powerful fibers that contain type 2 myosin.

Since type II fibers generate 4-6 times more power per unit mass than their slower type I fibers, our body calls on these faster fibers when they're required for power. Thus, performing the concentric part of each exercise with a powerful push or pull not only helps develop a strong, powerful physique, but it counteracts the reduction in type II fibers that impairs mobility and increases the risk of falls and fractures with age.

As innocent as it sounds, these falls commonly send the elderly on a path to early death. By training strength and power with compound lifts, explosive contractions, and periodized workouts, we have a higher probability of executing the rapid force production necessary to prevent them.

Executing our concentric action with explosiveness can be so effective at recruiting fast-fibers that research continuously shows better type II development with lighter weights, compared to normal speed contraction and heavier loads. Which is an encouraging finding for the aging population that's looking to counteract muscle and fiber loss and may not possess significant strength. As it suggests that the intent to execute the concentric movement with speed or maximal force, makes the amount lifted somewhat irrelevant.

> In a study from 2005 in the Journal of Gerontology, the greatest improvements in muscle power for older adults was found using 50% of 1RM and training with an explosive push or pull.

In other words, you can develop power without selecting max weights and sacrificing your form (so there's no point in killing yourself). Realistically, you're better off selecting a lighter load, or sacrificing a few reps, but achieving a maximum contraction.

Slow ECC + Fast CON = Optimal

As we just discussed, slower tempos extend the tension duration of an exercise (TUT), and this is superior for muscle development. For example, a study from 2006 in the Journal of Applied Physiology compared a 3 second eccentric and concentric tempo on a leg extension exercise with a lighter weight (50% 1RM) to a 1 second eccentric and concentric tempo with a heavier weight (80% 1RM). The slower tempo group had better muscle development over 12 weeks than the fast tempo group, despite much lighter weights!

However, we also learned that slower concentric actions are inferior to faster concentric actions for strength and muscle development. For instance, a study from 1993 in the Journal of Strength & Conditioning Research, split 18 male subjects into 2 groups, where one performed a controlled eccentric and fast concentric tempo in the squat (slow:fast) and the other performed a controlled tempo for both the eccentric and concentric part of the movement (slow:slow). Even though the results were very close (3.9% vs. 3.2%) the slow:fast group had better gains in muscle development than the slow:slow group. And not surprisingly, double the gains in force development (68.7% vs. 23.5%)!

Clearly, the slow eccentric and fast concentric tempo gives us everything we're looking for.

- A controlled TUT to benefit from the elevated metabolic stress and protein synthesis that promotes hypertrophy.
- More time spent in the eccentric action for greater strength and muscle development.

- The ability to perform the concentric action with speed to stimulate type-II muscle fiber action.
- No sacrifice in mechanical tension in an effort to increase metabolic stress.

Sadly, lifting too fast is extremely common. Not only because of the desire to lift heavier weight and crank out extra reps, but because our body and brain naturally want to speed up this stressful uncomfortable process.

> When you're not lifting with the proper speed, you're not training for the appropriate goal.

This is the reason the rest periods are different in the *1% Fitness* chart. Because even though we're seeking full muscle recovery between sets in both instances, strength reps require additional time for neurological recovery. Basically, we need our nervous system firing at all cylinders to push heavier weights, or we sacrifice performance on the upcoming set.

Optimal Recovery

Along with TUT, rest is critical in determining your results, as it has a significant impact on the metabolic and hormonal response to resistance training. Unfortunately, it's also the variable most commonly neglected.

> In general, shorter rest periods produce a larger hormonal response and more metabolic stress, while longer rest periods allow for more weight to be lifted on subsequent sets.

This is the reason the rest periods are different in the *1% Fitness* chart. Even though we're seeking full muscle recovery between sets in both instances, strength reps require additional time for neurological recovery. We need our nervous system firing at all cylinders to push heavier weights, or we sacrifice performance on the upcoming set.

	Set Range	Rep Range	Tempo	Total Rest
Strength	3 - 4	4 - 8	3010	2min or 60/60
Muscle	3 - 4	8 - 12	4010	1min or 30/30

What many fail to recognize, is that there's also a minimum rest threshold for hypertrophy (or muscle building) training. Yes, metabolic stress is one of the main drivers of hypertrophy, but we still need to recover between sets during 'muscle workouts.' As if rest periods are too short, the number of reps declines, the weight lifted declines, and so does the total workout volume. And any increase in metabolic stress is balanced by decreases in the other factors that trigger growth.

In other words, muscles swollen with exercise by-products and growth hormone are great for stimulating hypertrophy, but it's counterproductive if total volume and work load are sacrificed.

> A 2013 review published in the journal Sports Medicine analyzing research on hypertrophy, concluded that rest periods longer than 1 minute are preferable for maintaining optimal workloads while maintaining some metabolic stress.

We don't want the rest period at a point where it's difficult to perform as much as 'work' as would be possible with slightly longer rest. Which means keeping our rest between 90-120 seconds to maximize the number of successful reps over multiple sets while still experiencing adequate metabolic stress to stimulate hypertrophy. Anything below that (90 seconds), and we're effectively turning strength training into endurance training.

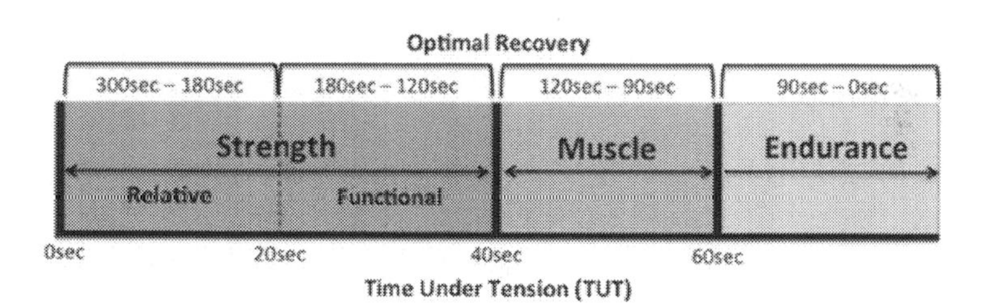

The reason many aspiring trainees never reach their goals, is because they mess up their recovery time. Generally, they can't put on muscle because their rest is too long, or they can't put on strength because their rest is too short. As you can see from the chart above, the magic happens between 90 and 180sec of recovery between sets. This maximizes hypertrophy (metabolic stress) without sacrificing strength (mechanical tension) on the low end, and maximizes strength without minimizing hypertrophy on the high end. Plus, it maximizes muscle-building hormones (testosterone, IGF-1, gH), with high volume and intensity, while minimizing the muscle-burning hormones (cortisol) associated with excessively short rest periods.

Combined vs. Split Rest

A notable point with respect to the rest column in the *1% Fitness* chart is that the values correspond to the upper-lower superset, NOT a strength or hypertrophy exercise on it's own. The 1-minute break for muscle-workouts and 2-minute break for strength-workouts is after performing a lower body exercise and an upper body exercise back to back.

	Set Range	Rep Range	Tempo	Total Rest
Strength	3 - 4	4 - 8	3010	2min or 60/60
Muscle	3 - 4	8 - 12	4010	1min or 30/30

The reason we're able to get into the 'optimal recovery' is because the seconds executing the one exercise count as total rest after the other exercise. For example, after completing the 1st set of the DB Goblet Squat in the workout below, the total recovery before the 2nd set of the DB Goblet Squat is 110-120 seconds.

	Exercise	Sets	Reps	Tempo	Rest
A1	DB Goblet Squat	4	10-12	4010	0sec
A2	Seated Pulldown	4	10-12	4010	60sec

Here's the math:

50-60 seconds performing the Seated Pulldown [10-12 (4+0+1+0)]

+

60 seconds rest after performing the Seated Pulldown

The other notable point is that you have a 30/30 and 60/60 option, as opposed to 1 or 2 minutes. Which means splitting the rest so we take 30 or 60 seconds after the lower body move, and 30 or 60 seconds after the upper body move.

Here's an example of both options with a strength-workout:

Option 1: Combined Rest

	Exercise	**Sets**	**Reps**	**Tempo**	**Rest**
A1	Incline DB Bench	4	6-8	3010	0sec
A2	45-degree Back Ext	4	6-8	3010	120sec

Option 2: Split Rest

	Exercise	**Sets**	**Reps**	**Tempo**	**Rest**
A1	Incline DB Bench	4	6-8	3010	60sec
A2	45-degree Back Ext	4	6-8	3010	60sec

In all of the *1% Fitness* workouts, you're given the option to rest after each exercise or perform your exercises back-to-back and rest longer. This can come in handy as a variety of factors can affect your workouts; like whether you train in a busy gym, and the intensity of each superset.

Adequate Volume

When we use the word 'volume' in resistance training, we mean the total number of sets multiplied by the total number of repetitions.

Workout Volume = Total Sets x Total Reps

Generally speaking, when the rep ranges are higher, the number of sets is lower; and visa versa. For instance, 3 sets would be most appropriate for a 10-rep protocol, and 5 sets for a 5-rep protocol.

Going back to our *1% Fitness* chart, a set range is provided to show you that we will be progressing from lower sets per exercise in the early phases (3), to higher set routines (4) as you improve.

	Set Range	**Rep Range**	**Tempo**	**Total Rest**
Strength	3 - 4	4 - 8	3010	2min or 60/60
Muscle	3 - 4	8 - 12	4010	1min or 30/30

Since we're working with 4 exercises in the upper-lower superset, and 1 core exercise to finish, this works out to 15 sets total (3 sets per exercise) on the low-end, and 20 sets total on the high-end (4 sets per exercise). Aside from being aligned with the current recommendations, experience with personal training clients over the last decade has led me to believe that this is the optimal workload for most individuals. Anything beyond that is likely excessive and unnecessary for the majority.

If you're an athlete or training to become a bodybuilder, I suggest seeking professional advice after building your baseline strength with *1% Fitness*. Both the majority of you reading this will be fine with the progression to 20 sets in Phase, as we're simply looking to build some strength and muscle, and live a longer, healthier life. Once we've reached this volume, we'll continue to maintain it, as 20 sets appears to be the ideal volume to maximize performance without over-training. Provided of course, that you're abiding by the rest, and selecting the appropriate weight for the given rep range and tempo.

Unlike the discrepancies surrounding rep ranges, the evidence supporting multiple sets over single-sets for muscle growth is quite substantial. We see superior elevations in muscle protein synthesis, and higher levels of hypertrophy when multiple sets are performed. Largely because more sets means more metabolic stress and greater overall workout volume.

> In a meta-analysis from 2010 in the Journal Strength & Conditioning Research, it was determined that multiple sets produce a 40% greater improvement in muscle hypertrophy compared to single sets (irrespective of training level or age).

There's also a sizeable difference in anabolic hormones (testosterone, growth hormone) in response to high-volume resistance training, when compared to low-volume.

> One study from 1993 in the journal Medicine & Science in Sports & Exercise found that testosterone did not rise until the 4th set on a squat workout.

And multiple set programs have even proven superior for strength, in both experienced and inexperienced individuals. While single-set training (1 set per exercise), on the other hand, has actually shown reductions in strength.

Frequent Variation to Avoid Stagnation

Once our body has adapted to a new stressor, there's less to be gained by applying it. We start recruiting less muscle mass to perform the same movement, and less strength and muscle is gained. Predominantly because this first adaptation was a form of survival, and the next time around it's less of a 'threat.'

In order to continuously progress we need to overload our muscles with a foreign stimulus. The obvious solution is increasing the weight, but this doesn't last forever. We eventually plateau (hit a strength peak) in a given exercise, and need to stress the muscles in a different way to improve. Which means changing any or all of the program variables listed below, to avoid the diminishing returns (drop off) in performance beyond the peak.

- Exercise selection (squat vs. lunge)
- Resistance choice (pulley vs. dumbbell)
- Exercise order (shoulder press at the start vs. at the end of the workout)
- Number of sets and reps
- Rest period length
- Repetition speed (tempo)
- Frequency (sessions per week)

In Strength Coach world, this is often referred to as Periodization. Unfortunately, it's another one of the things that can get confusing.

In a nutshell, you don't want to always be working to build muscle, or always be looking to build strength. Just like, you don't want to always be doing the same squat type, grip position, or pressing angle.

> Research suggests that loading variety is the key to long-term development in strength and muscle.

Instead of over-complicating things, we prevent plateaus in *1% Fitness* by moving back and forth between strength and muscle building workouts, and changing the exercises on each transition. Interestingly, (other than frequency) this simple muscle-strength swap takes care of all the exercise variables we listed above.

We're effectively applying two types of progression to avoid stagnation. Progression within a workout via reps and weight, and progression between workouts via the variables just listed. This plateau avoidance is essential to achieving a higher level of muscular fitness, as it affects the metabolic, hormonal, neural, and cardiovascular responses to resistance exercise.

> Whether male or female, experienced or inexperienced, old or young, research has proven that strength and hypertrophy gains are superior when exercises are consistently varied.

As you'll discover, we will be performing each workout 4 times before switching to a new set of exercises. Meaning 4 chances to get stronger, followed by 4 chances to build muscle. This consistent back and forth not only prevents plateau's, optimizes performance, and ensures adequate recovery, but it keeps thing exciting.

"There are many ways to skin a cat."

When your training goal is simply 'get strong and build muscle,' this strength-to-muscle-to-strength-to-muscle periodization plan, and consistent exercise variation is more than effective. Sure, you can come up with extremely elaborate periodization plans, that have you peaking for your 1 rep max bench press exactly 18 weeks from now. But, unless you're an Olympic athlete, what's the point?

Pausing during lifts (ex: 3110), doing light-weight high-rep sets (ex: 25), and grouping 3 exercises for the same muscle in a row are all great, but more than 15 years of experimentation, and nearly 10 years of hands-on experience with personal training clients, has led me to the *1% Fitness* chart below:

	Set Range	**Rep Range**	**Tempo**	**Total Rest**
Strength	3 - 4	4 - 8	3010	2min or 60/60
Muscle	3 - 4	8 - 12	4010	1min or 30/30

I've determined that this is the easiest way to learn, best way to execute, and most effective way to get the results you're looking for in the shortest commitment time possible. This method has proven itself in the past, and continues to deliver in the present.

I like simple, efficient, and effective; and since you're reading my book, I'm guessing you do too. If you push yourself with the variables provided in the *1% Fitness* charts, you will continue to gain strength and muscle.

"Winners compare their achievements with their goals, while losers compare their achievements with those of other people."

— Nido Qubein

Seek Progression Not Perfection (Lift Light, Get it Right)

After completing Phase 1, and learning the strategy for Phase 2, you're probably realizing that this is a 'progressive resistance training' plan. We're starting out with basic bodyweight exercises, adding weight to these movements, and then introducing more challenging progressions.

Though exercise selection is a very important piece of progressive resistance training, it's not the most critical component. One of the biggest factors in determining whether or not you experience the results you're pursuing is the consistent increase in weight. 'Progress' is the key word in progressive resistance training, and a conscious and consistent effort towards it, with incremental increases in weight, is the key to achieving it.

Don't get me wrong, you will see some changes by going from not lifting weights to lifting weights, but you'll eventually plateau without a consistent progression in weight.

> "In order to stimulate further adaptation toward specific training goals, progressive resistance training protocols are necessary." American College of Sports Medicine, 2009

Small Short-Term Increases = Big Long-Term Results

The best part about progression, is that from a workout-to-workout perspective, the weight increases are minimal. You simply try to improve on your last performance in a given exercise, whether that's adding 5lbs to the bar, moving to the dumbbells that are 2.5lbs heavier, or getting 10 reps on set 2, when you only got 8 reps on set 2 last week.

The principle says "Seek Progression NOT Perfection," for a reason. You don't get a chizzled physique or double your bench press or squat overnight. Like most things, it takes time. All you can do is keep pushing for small jumps in weight, or reps, with each workout.

As we discussed in Principle #6, you're supplied with a given rep range at each exercise and the goal is to choose a weight that's challenging within that range. For example, if you were asked to complete 8-10 reps on a Flat Dumbbell Bench Press, you'd want to choose a weight that you could do for 8, 9, or 10 reps. And generally speaking:

> *If you can't do the lower number (ex: 8) in the rep range, the weight is too heavy.*
>
> *If you're getting the higher number (ex: 10) with ease, the weight is too light.*

There's obviously a bit of trial and error here, as failing to get 8 reps on set 1 isn't the same as failing to get 8 reps on set 3. And getting 10 reps with ease on set 3 is a lot different than getting 10 reps with ease on set 1. But in a nutshell, that's the guideline.

Here's an example:

Scenario 1: 10 reps with ease on Set 1

	Set 1	**Set 2**	**Set 3**
Flat DB Bench	25 - 10 reps	25 – 9 reps	25 – 8 reps

Scenario 2: 10 reps with ease on Set 3

	Set 1	**Set 2**	**Set 3**
Flat DB Bench	25 - 10 reps	25 – 10 reps	25 – 10 reps

In Scenario 2, set 3 for 10 reps was easy, so increasing the weight next workout would be encouraged.

In Scenario 1, set 1 for 10 reps was easy, but set 2 and 3 were challenging (only 9 reps and 8 reps were completed), so keeping the weight the same next workout and working to get 10 reps at all 3 sets would be encouraged.

Here's another example:

Scenario 1: Failing to get 8 reps on Set 1

	Set 1	**Set 2**	**Set 3**
Flat DB Bench	25 - 7 reps	20 – 10 reps	20 – 9 reps

Scenario 2: Failing to get 8 reps on Set 3

	Set 1	**Set 2**	**Set 3**
Flat DB Bench	25 – 9 reps	25 – 8 reps	25 – 7 reps

In Scenario 1, 25lbs was too heavy for 8 reps, so the trainee dropped the weight to 20lbs to stay in the proper rep range (8-10 reps). Continuing at 25lbs would have been a mistake.

In Scenario 2, the trainee was in the rep range on set 1 and 2, but failed to get 8 on the final set. If there was a 4th set, lowering the weight to 20lbs would make sense, but because there were only 3 sets, this was perfect. The correct move when attempting this workout again (in scenario 2) would be to keep the weight at 25lbs, until 10 reps can be completed at all 3 sets with ease.

To reiterate, the goal is to choose a weight that challenges you in the given rep range. If you are not hitting the lower number in the range, it's too heavy. If you are consistently hitting the upper number with ease, it's too light. When it comes to reps, this is the backbone of progressive resistance training.

> Steadily increasing weight (or reps) each time a workout is repeated, is the key to experiencing continuous improvements in strength and muscle.

Most studies recommend anywhere from a 2-10% increment once you can perform a selected weight with ease. Which could be as small as a 2.5lb or 5lb increase from your previous session.

Honestly, it's surprising how much progress you can make in a given workout with minimal increases from a workout-to-workout basis. As an example, let's say one of Jim's workouts has him doing Flat Dumbbell Bench Press for 4 sets of 6-8 reps. And these are his numbers after completing the exercise 4 separate times over 2 weeks:

Exercise	**Sets x Reps**	**Reps/Weight**
Flat DB Bench	4 x 6-8	45/8,45/8,50/7,50/6
		50/8,50/7,50/7,50/6
		50/8,50/8,50/8,50/8
		50/8,55/7,55/6,50/8

Jim managed to climb from 45lbs for 8 reps to nearly 55lbs for 8 reps, which is a considerable amount of progress over 4 sessions. Especially, when you consider that 10lbs per dumbbell equates to 20lbs overall; or a 22% increase!

Even more outstanding, is when you add that single-workout progress over time. Sure, it won't be 22% with every workout, but even 5-10% improvement every 2 weeks adds up quickly.

For untrained individuals, the jumps in performance will be much larger; especially at first. This is partly because of inexperience with the movements and getting familiar with lifting weights in general, but it's also because of the tendency to choose weights that are too light for the given rep range. As knowingly or not, research has determined that we subconsciously self-select weights or intensities that are lower than what is recommended.

Slow to Grow

The only thing that discourages an increase in weight or reps is sloppy form or an improper tempo.

Execution (Form & Tempo) > Performance (Weight & Reps)

As you learned in Principle #6, the speed of the lift is essential to reaching the suitable Time Under Tension (TUT) for your training goal. When you lift weight too fast you end up training for strength instead of muscle, displacing the other exercise variables (rest, rep range) and messing with the periodization plan.

Unfortunately, this is extremely common, as it's natural to think more weight means more muscle. Even though we gain a lot more when we slow it down and extend the TUT. For instance, take a look at a 1-5 rep protocol and compare it to 6-12 reps. Although it's often debated which one is better or worse for muscle building, there's more evidence pointing to 6-12 as the superior range for muscle building.

Why?

Because the TUT is higher! When the muscle is under tension longer we use anaerobic glycolysis system, which results in a build-up of metabolites that have a considerable impact on anabolic factors. Even though less reps and shorter tension periods give us the ability to lift heavier weights, the concentration of blood and lactate, and elevations in testosterone and gH (muscle building hormones), are significantly larger with higher rep ranges.

Just take a look at the way bodybuilders train, and the way powerlifters train. A bodybuilder stresses his muscles by keeping them under tension for extended periods of time and overloading them with lactate, blood, and other metabolites. This swelling and stress-induced response (also known as 'the pump') is what stimulates adaptation and growth.

The powerlifter, on the other hand, performs his repetitions explosively and takes longer recovery periods because his main priority is strength. Yes, the powerlifter lifts a lot more weight, but the bodybuilder is a lot bigger. And sure, the powerlifter can gain muscle, as mechanical tension and overload are contribute to hypertrophy (muscle growth), but he'd gain a lot more if he slowed it down (like the bodybuilder) and generated higher levels of metabolic stress – the biggest muscle building factor.

For the record, this doesn't mean you'll look like a big bodybuilder by training with a slower tempo (ladies!). We're not doing nearly enough volume, and you have nowhere near the testosterone for that. It also doesn't mean we won't put on strength (guys!). We'll gain considerable strength in the 4-12 rep range, and continue to progress if we're increasing the weight at each workout.

Lift Light, Get it Right

Aside from aligning our training zone with our training goal, controlling our tempo prevents current and future injuries by forcing us to think about form and execute movements properly.

Most people work with weights that are too heavy, which causes them to lift improperly, and set themselves up for injury.

Starting with a lighter weight and working our way up is critical, especially when it's a brand new workout or exercise. This does require checking our ego at the door, but executing these lifts properly makes the remainder of our lifting career go off without a hitch. Muscles have a memory, so it's essential that we perfect our movement patterns from the start.

If we flip back and look at the scenarios from earlier, our decision on whether or not to increase the weight next time around would depend on how our 10 reps was performed.

Scenario 1: 10 reps with ease on Set 1

	Set 1	**Set 2**	**Set 3**
Flat DB Bench	25 - 10 reps	25 – 9 reps	25 – 8 reps

Scenario 2: 10 reps with ease on Set 3

	Set 1	**Set 2**	**Set 3**
Flat DB Bench	25 - 10 reps	25 – 10 reps	25 – 10 reps

With Scenario 1, your decision to attempt 27.5lbs or 30lbs next time doing this workout, would depend on how well you executed your 10, 9, and 8 rep sets. Sloppy form or a quick tempo may mean staying at 25lbs for all sets. Spectacular form and perfect tempo may mean trying to hit 27.5lbs on set 2 after a clean set 1 for 10.

For those concerned with muscular strength, don't be. Research has shown that it can still be improved using weights that are less than 65% of full strength in untrained individuals. Likewise, increases in the markers for hypertrophy (like muscle protein synthesis) have been equivalent with lighter weights (30% of full strength) performed to failure, compared to heavier weights (80-90%) to failure.

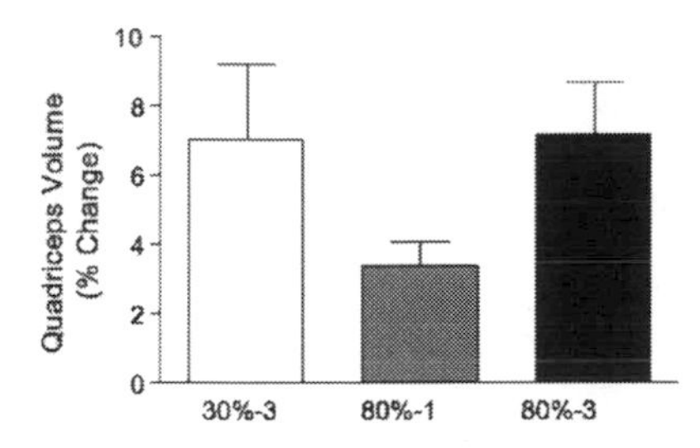

In other words, if you're a beginner, lifting lighter weights and learning the form will not prevent you from developing. You will still gain strength and muscle by choosing weights you're comfortable lifting for the given repetition range.

Unfortunately, that does change with training age; as the load required for development appears to be associated with training experience. However, by the time you'll need to lift 80% or more of your 1RM (rep max) to make additional gains, you'll have plenty of experience to feel comfortable with it.

Lifting right also means performing the exercise to full range of motion. Unless stated otherwise, all of the exercises in *1% Fitness* call for a maximum stretch of the muscle followed by a full contraction. Looking at the Flat Dumbbell Bench Press for example, this means bringing the weight to a full shoulder and pec stretch in the bottom position, and locking out the elbows completely at the top. Aside from increasing flexibility and helping prevent injuries, this leads to a more physically appealing, maximally muscled physique.

> A 2013 in the European Journal of Applied Physiology compared half squats (0-60 degrees) vs. full squats (0-120 degrees) in 24 young male subjects, and found significantly greater increases in all areas of the front thigh for the full squat group.

If you have an injury preventing you from going full range, get it fixed! This is not an injury treatment program, it's an injury prevention program. You can still work on perfecting the lifestyle factors and building on the bodyweight movements from Phase 1, but please avoid jumping into weight-bearing movements until you're ready. There's a reason, standing tall, sitting less, walking and squatting daily, rebuilding your feet, and getting strong in your own skin are part of Phase 1. And there's a reason *Live It NOT Diet!* is the pre-requisite to *1% Fitness*. No disrespect, but go back and get fixed up and come join us in Phase 2 when you're lean, flexible, strong, balanced, and healthy.

Match Breathing to Tempo

One of the most challenging things for new weight-trainees to grasp is proper breathing. Aside from the fact that they already have way too many things to think about, there's a natural tendency to breathe backwards. For whatever reason, it's very common to breath in on the concentric or explosive part of the lift, when you should be breathing out. Through trial and error with clients, I've determined that the easiest way to nail your breathing is to think:

Slow & In - Fast & Out

In other words, take a slow deep breath in during the controlled or eccentric part of the lift (big number – 4 or 3), and a fast short breath out during the explosive or concentric part (small number – 1). Breathing in longer keeps oxygen coming in, and blowing out fast on the push pull helps propel the weight with force.

When looking at thc Flat Dumbbell Bench Press, you'd breathe in slow while lowering the weights to your chest for 3 or 4 seconds, and breathe out fast when pressing the weight back up.

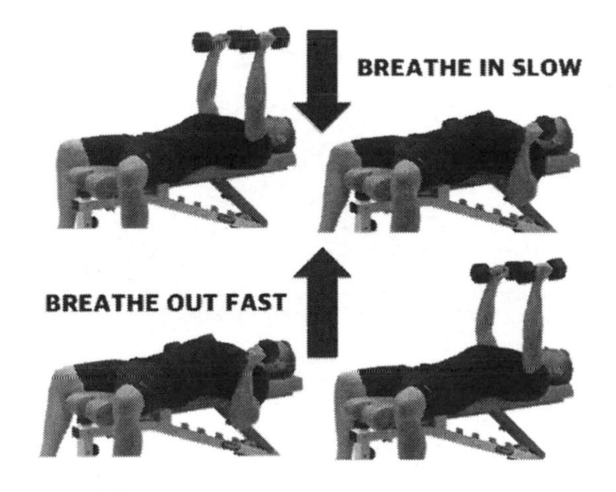

The same rule holds true for pulling movements, but as you'll discover, it's the opposite with respect to the positioning of the bar when breathing in or out. Unlike the press, the 'in' is when you're extending the arms, and the 'out' is when you're bringing the bar closer.

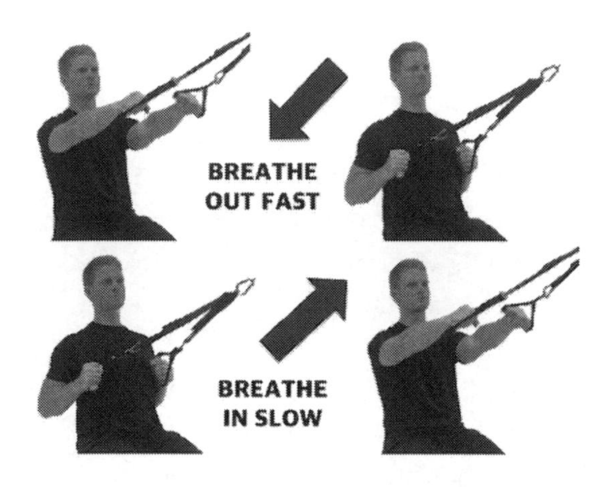

Although pulling can be a confusing time for clients, nothing changes with respect to our 'Slow & In, Fast & Out' rule. Since the eccentric (slow) part of a pull is when your arms extend away from your body, this is when you breathe in. And since the concentric (fast) part is when you pull the weight close to your body, this is when you breathe out.

Similar to the various opinions on tempo's, and rep and set schemes, there are different breathing options that have proven beneficial. However, they only appear to be helpful during very heavy lifting. And like I said before, they're unnecessary unless you're an extremely advanced lifter.

As far as I'm concerned, 'Slow In & Fast Out' is all you need to succeed. I've been doing it for 15 years, and aside from advantageously holding my breath at times to squeak out more difficult reps, I've never looked back.

Intensity = Lift More Weight NOT Lift Weight More

Other than the word functional, 'intensity' is one of the most misunderstood terms in fitness. I know you're picturing a sweaty out-of-breath person that could run to the bathroom and puke at any moment, because we've been taught to associate intensity with exhaustion.

> *Who knows, maybe this is also why we think 'cardio' is the best exercise choice?*

When we speak about intensity in *1% Fitness*, we mean pushing our muscles to their maximum capacity within the designated training variables. Which means choosing a weight that's optimal for the given rep range (not too light or heavy) and executing the movement with the proper form and tempo. If the form and tempo is not there, the weight is too heavy, or exercise choice too challenging. The proper reaction is lowering the load, or regressing to an easier variation of the movement. Conversely, if the form and tempo are clean, and you're not challenged on the final rep, raise the weight.

Along with continuously progressing to more challenging weights within the designated workout parameters, rest is going to determine the intensity of the workout. Again, this is not 'exhaustion' or 'depletion,' this is intensity. Yes, you may be slightly out of breath, and yes blood will be pumping through your muscles, but this is different than aerobic fitness. We're not tiring you to the point where you can't do anything, we're working your muscles to their maximum capacity, and giving them adequate rest to stay strong.

This requires being strict with the rest periods in the *1% Fitness* chart, and looking to progress within the other parameters.

Unfortunately, our obsession with exhaustive training also has us believing that we should be exercising continuously. "No Rest for the Wicked" is what Aerobic Instructors and Cardio Kings will tell you. And sadly, even many CrossFitters and High-Intensity Circuit Trainers seemed to have transitioned to the dark side, with their "No Pain, No Gain" mantra.

It's all about Muscle Confusion right?

I'm not here to bash other training methods, but any qualified fitness professional understands that the work-to-rest ratio determines the training zone. And if we work too long, or rest too short, we start training a different energy system.

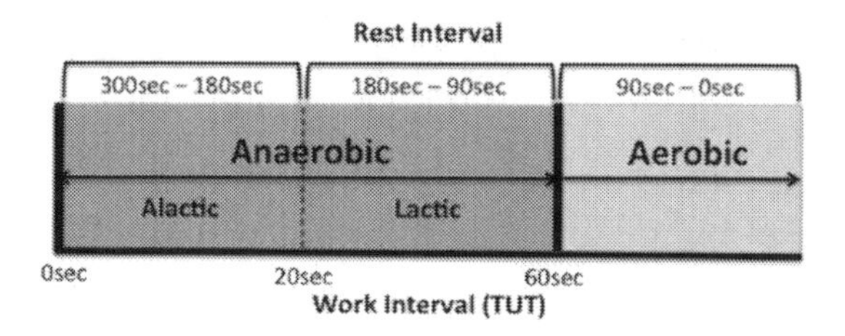

We're not trying to exhaust the muscle, we're trying to strengthen and improve it. When we perform an endless number of muscle contractions (repetitions), we end up building muscular endurance as opposed to hypertrophy or strength. Training the muscle aerobically, instead of anaerobically.

Aside from accelerating the muscle loss and fiber shift that's associated with aging, this decreases our overall power and explosiveness. The very thing we're looking to BUILD, not burn!

Raise Intensity Not Duration or Frequency

You can bring intensity to *1% Fitness*, but it's not achieved by doing things faster or longer. Bringing intensity is nailing your rest, and selecting a challenging weight that you can perform with perfect form and tempo. Don't shorten the rest, or do extra sloppy reps, like the exhausted exerciser. And don't do partial reps with a weight that's too heavy, or take 5 minutes between sets like a bro with an ego. The best way to prove yourself is to make consistent gains week after week within the workout parameters provided. That's the true definition of 'bringing intensity' to your workouts.

If I was there, I'd be happy to see you start your set when your timer goes off, only get 7 reps on a set of 8-10, and lower the weight the following set. I'd also be excited to see you fatiguing with a light-weight and a really strict tempo on your last set.

Likewise, I'd be disappointed to see extended rest periods and accelerated tempos. As sure you'd get some results, but nothing like what you could achieve if you rested properly and chose the optimal weight.

The same principle applies to the frequency of your training. Although you may feel like you have the energy to add a 3rd session before phase 3, I suggest using it to focus on walking more, sitting less, and working on the other lifestyle factors that improve your health and body composition. Realistically, you're better off bottling up that extra intensity and looking to consistently progress during your 2 lifting sessions.

Frankly, the ones looking to 'work out more' fall into 2 categories. Group 1 coasts through workouts with weights that are too light, tempo's that are too fast, and rest periods that are too long. Group 2 eats like crap, and is convinced they can out-exercise their mistakes. In both cases, more exercise is not the solution.

Rest Determines Result

The goal of resistance training is to overload the body so it can adapt in a positive way; which can come in the form of more strength and muscle, or improvements in insulin sensitivity and muscle protein synthesis. But when exercise is excessive - usually because of inadequate rest – these improvements are compromised, and can lead to injury and muscle loss.

Just as there's extreme exercise in the form of cardiovascular training, people often beat themselves into the ground with weight training. As we discussed in *Eat Meat And Stop Jogging*, 'more' is not always 'better' when it comes to exercise; and one of the reasons for that is because of the stress hormone cortisol.

Research from 2012 in the Journal of Strength and Conditioning Research found extremely high cortisol and lactate levels following a pyramid style (10 sets of 10 reps down to 1) bench press, deadlift, and squat workout with no rest. The workout was so stressful, that cortisol levels ended up being higher than what was typically seen after high-intensity interval or traditional cardiovascular training. And although they returned to baseline the next day, one could expect to see the same catabolic (muscle loss) environment and poor T:C ratio experienced with aerobic training, if this type of protocol was taken part in several times a week. As the researchers put it:

> "this has potentially serious implications on muscle tissue growth, recovery, and immune processes due to the catabolic effects of cortisol."

Whether it's resistance training or not.

Interestingly, 'overtraining' is usually the result of too much volume, not too much intensity. Thus, trying to work out more 'often' does not always lead to better results; it simply makes us tired, unmotivated, and prone to getting sick or injured.

Fortunately, the workouts in *1% Fitness* are designed to keep muscle building hormones high, and muscle-wasting hormones low. The controlled tempos, challenging free-weight compound movements, consistent progression in weight, and short rest periods will keep intensity high throughout the workout, within an optimal training duration of 20-30 minutes. Plus, our back-and-forth between muscle and strength phases, and 2-day recovery between lifts will optimize performance and recovery.

But you can do your part by focusing on improving your daily low-intensity activity, and aligning your lifestyle with your primal past. Walk, sit in a deep squat, rebuild your feet, and get plenty of sleep, because that's the secret to growth!

"All of the body's important recovery and adaptive processes require specific nutrients to proceed optimally. For this reason, the period immediately following a workout is the most important...from a nutritional perspective."

— Drs. John Ivy & Robert Portman

Do Post-Workout the Right 'Whey'

Throughout the course of the day, there's a balance between muscle protein synthesis (MPS) and muscle protein breakdown (MPB). Generally speaking, regular protein consumption stimulates MPS and slightly reduces MPB (positive protein balance), and fasting reduces MPS and slightly increases MPB (negative protein balance).

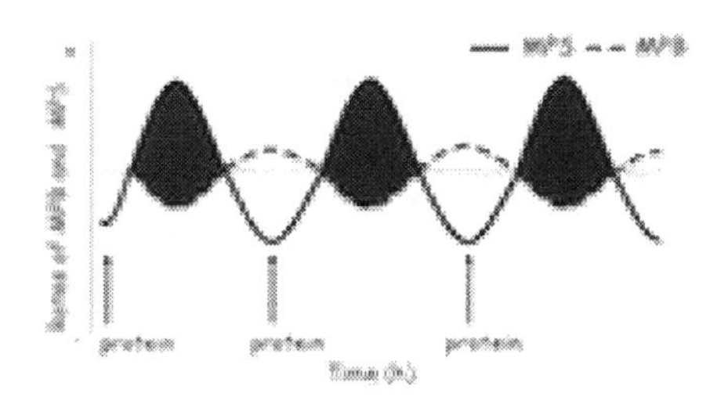

This is important, because muscle mass and hypertrophy is determined by the net balance between MPS and MPB.

> When MPS is elevated, proteins are manufactured at a faster rate, and there's an increased need and utilization of protein.

Fortunately, consuming protein rich foods high in essential amino acids is not the only way to stimulate MPS. The other way is with resistance training, and this is one of the reasons it's so critical for muscle.

What's interesting about the elevations in MPS after resistance training, is that they're not a measly old 3-4hr elevation like animal protein, but rather an increase that can last anywhere from 48-72hrs after a lifting session.

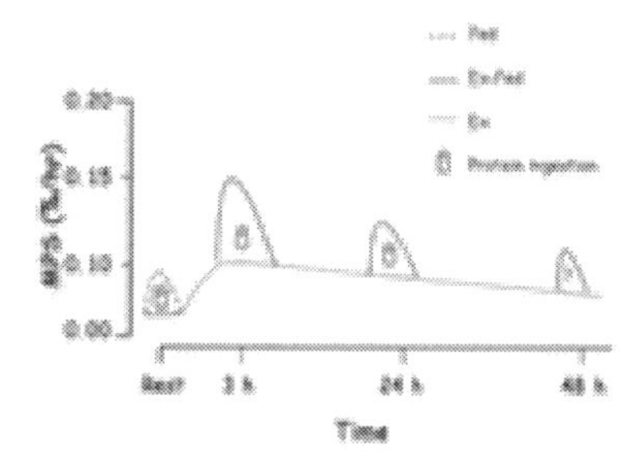

The best part is, we can enhance and extend this already elevated MPS window, and supress any potential muscle protein breakdown (MPB), by consuming protein after resistance training.

> "Nutritional strategies that serve to maximally stimulate MPS may be useful in the development of nutrition and exercise based interventions aimed at enhancing skeletal muscle mass which may be of interest to elderly populations and to athletes."

So, we don't consume protein after resistance training because we burned protein, as less than 2% is used during a session under 1 hour. We also don't consume it to prevent damage or enhance muscle recovery, as the most up-to-date research says there are no significant improvements in either of these measures. The main reason we consume protein after resistance training, is because it helps enhance muscle growth by elevating MPS.

The Best 'Whey' to Stimulate MPS

If you've completed *Live It NOT Diet!*, you understand that dairy is best consumed in it's full fat form. Mainly because that's where most of the benefit lies when dealing with the pasteurized variety we have access to. As the fat is all that seems to successfully survive the process of skimming, filtering, and heating.

The other reason we stick to full-fat dairy sources (heavy cream, aged cheeses, and butter) is because they contain minimal amounts of lactose and whey. Lactose is the sugar in dairy that a sizeable portion of the population has trouble breaking down, and whey is the liquid protein that gives us a ginormous insulin spike.

> Whey is capable of raising insulin levels more than table sugar and white bread!

You could say that whey is somewhat of a Friend & Foe, or Bittersweet Food. As clearly we should avoid it on a regular basis to stay lean, insulin sensitive, and disease-free, but it's also unique in its ability to stimulate MPS.

Although various types of dietary proteins (casein, beef, egg, etc.), can be beneficial following resistance training, they differ significantly in their capacity to stimulate protein synthesis. For instance, research consistently shows greater elevations following the consumption of whey and bovine milk compared to other proteins. Largely because it's rich in the essential amino acids (EAAs) that are critical for muscle growth.

Grams per 25g	**Whey**	**Casein**	**Soy**
EAA	12.4	11.0	9.0
BCAA	5.6	4.9	3.4
Leucine	3.0	2.3	1.5

EAAs have a significant impact on MPS, while non-essential amino acids have minimal if any impact. Leucine is mentioned in the chart above because it's the most critical. And aside from the other health benefits of whey (that we'll discuss shortly), it's high Leucine content is the reason it comes so highly recommended for post-workout nutrition.

Whey > Casein

As we discussed in *Live It NOT Diet!*, whey is the liquid protein in dairy that separates from the solid portion (casein) when making cheese. This composition makes the amino acids in whey instantly absorbed, and a superior post-workout beverage compared to milk products or casein protein (which coagulates in stomach acid).

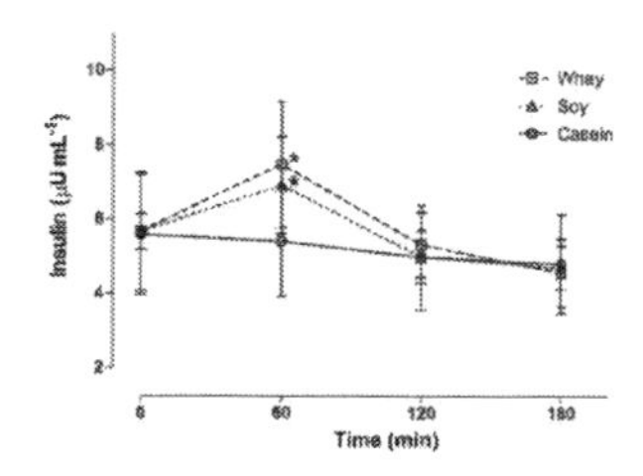

As the next two charts illustrate, this spike in insulin is largely driven by the amino acid and leucine content of whey.

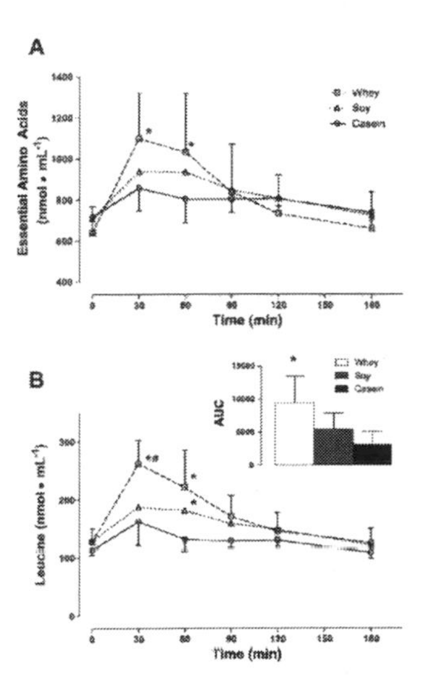

This small difference leads to anywhere from a 68-122% greater increase in muscle protein synthesis when consuming whey instead of casein after exercise.

When compared to soy, whey has a better amino acid profile profile and impact on MPS. However, there's no need to go into great detail with that, as we already discussed the problems with soy in *Eat Meat And Stop Jogging.*

> Soy is toxic to humans whether it's non-GMO, isoflavone-free, or whatever they're trying to sell it as.

And even if we forget the health consequences and look strictly at performance, soy decreases muscular strength, lowers testosterone and increases cortisol when consumed post-workout. The exact opposite of what we get from whey, and the exact opposite of what we need to live a longer stronger life.

Side Benefits of Whey

When it comes to dairy intolerance, we're more likely to be sensitive to casein or lactose than whey. As generally, the whey proteins (lactoferrin, albumin, and lactalbumin) are more easily digested by humans, as this is the predominant protein in breast milk (3:1). Compared to cow's milk, which is mostly casein (4:1).

Fortunately, whey is also where the immune protecting antibodies (IgA) are located, and the amino acids that support the production of an extremely important antioxidant. Several of the amino acids in whey protein (notably cysteine) help our body produce more glutathione, which helps counteract free radicals and reduce our risk of the diseases associated with oxidative damage. Despite being commonly blamed for allergic reactions, the glutathione supporting whey proteins (alpha-lacto albumin, beta-lacto globulin, lactoferrin, immune-globulin) in dairy have actually been shown to reduce eczema and asthma.

These glutathione producing properties are also why we see such an extensive list of health benefits attached to whey:

- Increasing serotonin and cognitive function
- Improving vitamin A absorption
- Inhibiting the growth of pathogenic bacteria (like E. coli)
- Reducing oxidative stress and neutralizing toxins
- Encouraging the growth of beneficial (probiotic) bacteria

- Protecting against tumor growth and reducing cancer risk
- Reducing liver fat
- Improving bone healing and preventing bone loss
- Increasing satiety and reducing food intake
- Improving fasting glucose and insulin sensitivity
- Elevating resting energy expenditure and fat oxidation
- Reducing heart disease risk – blood pressure, lipid profile, and vascular function
- Improving symptoms of autism and depression

Interestingly, the anti-cancer effects of whey protein seem to cancel out any cancer-promoting effects that have been attributed to casein. Suggesting that nature looks to protect us with the natural composition of whole foods (i.e. breast milk), and implying that if we're going to choose a powdered protein to consume, whey makes the most sense.

> *Note: Before you go inspecting the ingredients on all your full-fat dairy products, I should mention that the casein-cancer correlation has only been shown in rats at EXTREMELY high doses. Even if 20% of your diet consists of cheese, the increased risk of liver cancer is negligible. Plus, the research comes via the same vegan that did scientific gymnastics to bring us The China Study!*

Types of Whey – Concentrate, Isolate, Hydrosylate

For some, whey protein may seem expensive, but that's usually before comparing it serving-to-serving to meat. In most cities in North America, a decent quality chicken breast is going to cost upwards of $4-5 and only provide 20-25g of protein, while 1 scoop of whey is less than $2-3 and provides 25-30g of protein. More importantly, 25g of chicken breast does not have the same amino acid profile and resulting MPS elevation as 25g of whey.

In order to get the equivalent amount of leucine – the most critical amino acids for muscle building – you'd need to eat close to 50g of chicken breast!

When compared to a big plate of animal protein, a liquid protein like whey is digested quickly. Meaning amino acid absorption and MPS stimulation can happen almost instantly.

Where you can save money, is opting for a concentrate or isolate instead of hydrolysate. The bodybuilder at your local supplement shop may try to encourage you otherwise as hydrolysate is more quickly absorbed, and results in a larger insulin spike.

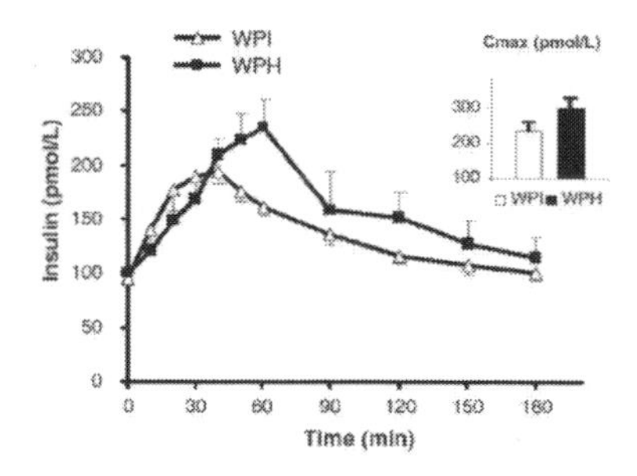

However, I'm not convinced the minimal superiority in MPS is worth the investment. Plus, the whey is exposed to intense heat to break apart the bonds linking the amino acids (pre-digest). Not only making it taste worse, but resulting in a reduction in the beneficial components we just discussed (beta-lacto globulin, etc.).

Maximal Health Increase > Minimal MPS Increase

Aside from its effect on MPS, the reason whey protein is highly recommended over other protein sources (casein, egg, soy, pea, rice, etc.) is because it increases glutathione, which supports our immune function. Unfortunately, it can only do this effectively in its raw un-pasteurized form, as beta-lactaglobulin and serum albumin are very sensitive to heat.

> A study from 1981 in the Journal of Agricultural and Food Chemistry exposed raw whey protein to both high-temperature short-time (HTST) and ultra-high temperature (UHT) pasteurization, and it resulted in 22% and 45% less beta-lacto globulin, respectively.

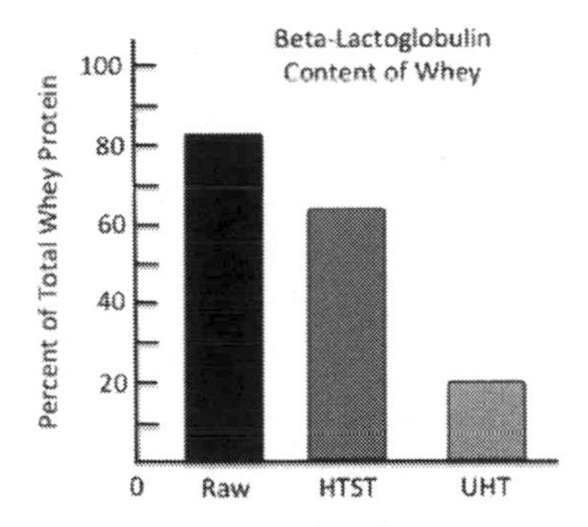

Likewise, a study from 2001 in the International Journal of Food Science & Technology showed that exposing raw dairy to HTST (65-85 degrees Celsius) reduces the serum albumin by 40-77%, and UHT almost destroys it completely.

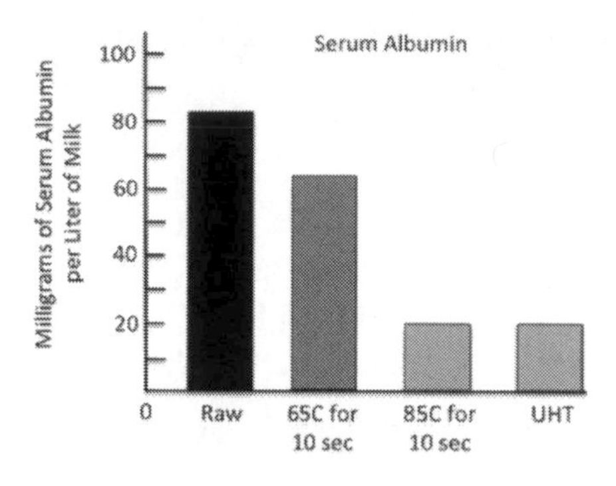

When looking at lactoferrin, raw milk was a whopping 2,866 times higher than boiled milk and a mind-blowing 8,026 times higher than UHT milk!

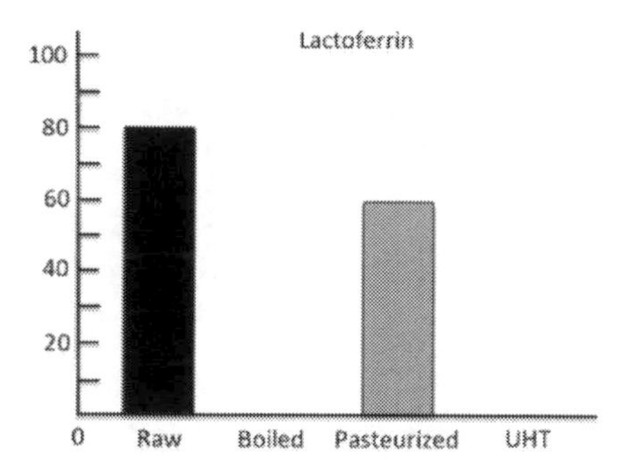

Fortunately for us, research suggests that beneficial glutathione production can still occur with standard pasteurization (around 60 degrees Celsius for 30 minutes), as the sensitive whey proteins are not nearly as negatively affected as they are under high-heat processing. Minimal pasteurization causes a much lesser loss of lactoferrin (36%), bovine serum albumin (56%), and beta-lacto globulin, compared to the way it's obliterated when boiled or put through HTST or UHT.

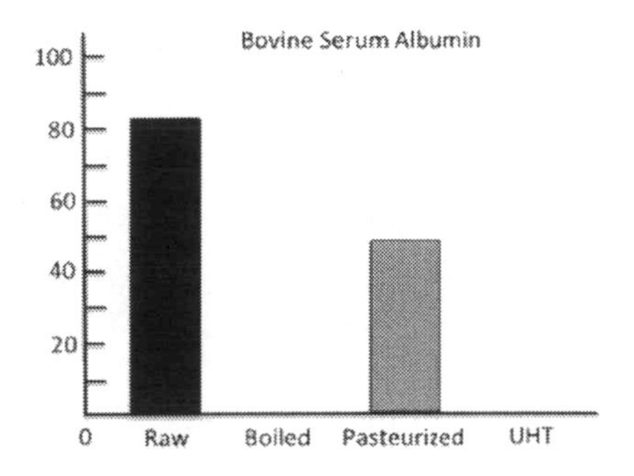

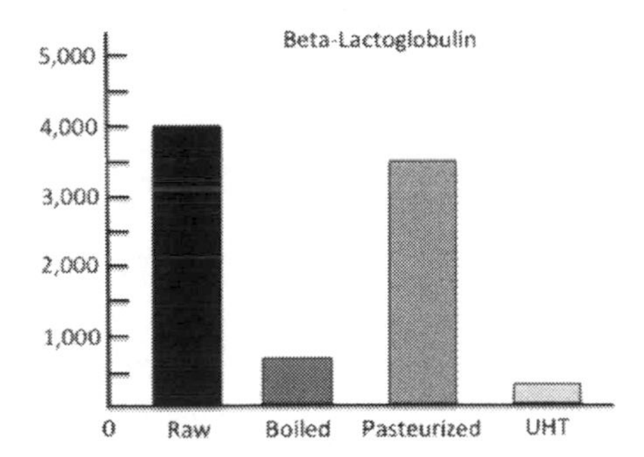

Obviously, your best bet is consuming whey in it's raw form, to get as much immune boosting support as possible; but in most cases, you'll have to settle with 'lightly-pasteurized' whey. In any case, I don't think the extra MPS from hydrolysate is worth the loss in glutathione boosting protein. Especially when you can get a minimally pasteurized whey concentrate or isolate for half the price!

Your decision to go concentrate or isolate comes down to how much you can spend, and whether you can handle sugar and lactose. Generally speaking, whey concentrate is closer to 'real food' as it is the actual liquid mixture leftover after separating from the solid casein during cheese production. Unfortunately, this means it comes with more carbs and lactose than a whey isolate, which is put through an extra step to 'isolate' the protein. So, for someone with a lot to lose, or a notable intolerance to lactose, paying more for this extra step is well worth it.

Interestingly, one could argue that it also makes sense for the rest of us, as we end up getting more grams of protein and amino acids per serving, and a significantly higher level of MPS.

With respect to immune-boosting benefits, scientists have developed a process to transform whey concentrate into whey isolate without adding heat - meaning glutathione production is unaffected. That being said, this is an important thing to look for when deciding whether or not to spend the extra money on an isolate. Similar to the way the pasteurization process is a key consideration when purchasing a concentrate.

> *It would be pretty foolish to choose concentrate over isolate to avoid denatured proteins, when the concentrate was pasteurized under the same high-heat.*

Of interest, most of the positive research cited earlier, used a whey protein isolate. Perhaps suggesting that there's no downside to choosing isolate over concentrate, other than price. Especially if we look for a minimally pasteurized, low- or no-heat treated product.

Optimal Dose of Whey

There appears to be an optimal dose of both leucine and whey. And any extra protein and amino acids beyond this dose have no additional impact on MPS and essentially go to waste. Something scientists have dubbed 'the muscle full effect.'

For example, in 2009 researchers in the American Journal of Clinical Nutrition found no additional elevations in MPS following the ingestion 40g of whey protein after resistance training, compared to 20g. The young men in the study simply oxidized the additional amino acids.

Knowing that the participants in the AJCN study all weighed approximately 86kg, it's clear that the optimal dose of whey falls somewhere between 0.23g and 0.46g per kg bodyweight. We also know that 20g of whey has approximately 2.5g of leucine, so the optimal dose of leucine is somewhere between 0.03g and 0.06g per kg bodyweight.

Other evidence on post-workout protein confirms these amounts, and steers us closer to 0.3g per kg of bodyweight for whey and 0.04g/kg of leucine. For an 80kg (176lb) man, this equates to a whey protein dose of 24g, and for a 60kg (132lb) women, this equates to a whey protein dose of approximately 18g.

Optimal Post-Workout Dose = 0.3g/kg bodyweight of whey protein

Ironically, the leucine content in this dose is almost exactly 0.04g/kg. Once again suggesting that nature is looking out for us.

Older? You May Need More Whey

We've already discussed some of the implications of aging. Including a 0.5-2% loss of muscle mass per year when there's no effort to gain and maintain it. This decline in muscle mass (sarcopenia) is largely driven by an impaired ability to increase protein production (MPS) in response to feeding and loading.

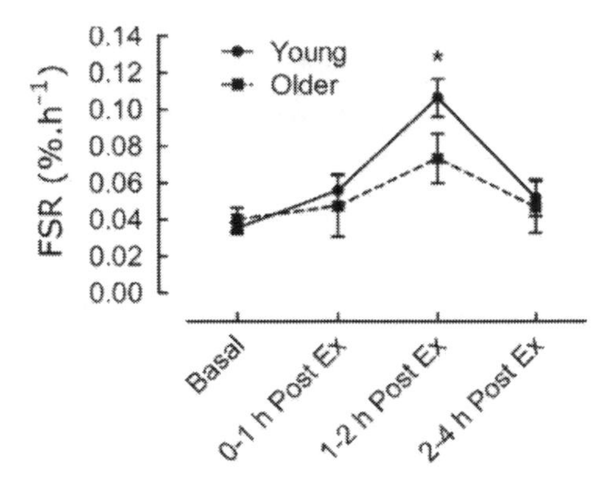

Similar to muscle loss, this 'anabolic resistance' is often classified as a normal consequence of aging. Even though just like muscle loss, it's more like a normal consequence of inactivity and poor nutrition.

For instance, research from 1985 in the journal of Applied Physiology found that:

> "the acute MPS response after resistance exercise and EAA ingestion is similar between young and old men; however, the response is delayed with aging."

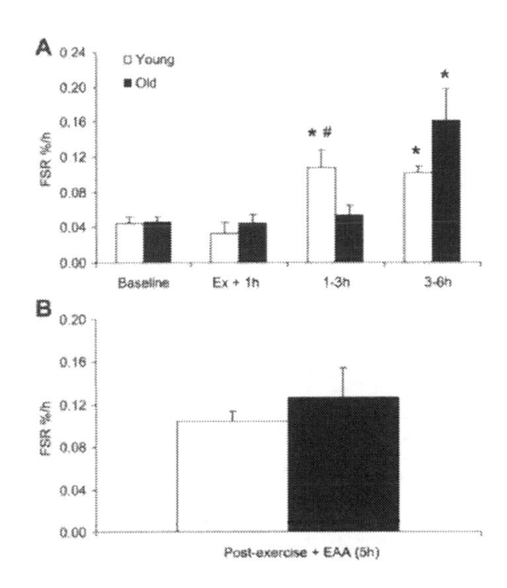

Note the difference between young and old in the 'Ex+1' column in the first chart above. The MPS marker was higher for the older muscle after resistance training, and the younger muscle didn't take over until the ingestion of protein and amino acids. Suggesting that old muscle is more than capable of stimulating MPS through resistance training and can improve the ability following protein ingestion by improving tissue sensitivity.

> Muscle cells become resistant when they lose receptor sites (inactivity + high-carb diet) and become sensitive when they gain receptor sites (resistance training + low-carb diet).

Fortunately, if you're already following *Live It NOT Diet!* you're ahead of the game. You'll continue to improve your insulin sensitivity, and maintain a proper balance between MPS and MPB throughout the day. The addition of resistance training and prioritization of post-workout nutrients will only enhance your tissue sensitivity, and work to combat the muscle loss associated with aging.

If you're not, or you just started the plan, you may benefit from slightly higher doses of post-workout protein. I wouldn't suggest going crazy with it, but increasing your bodyweight calculation dose to 0.5g/kg might be necessary to fully benefit from protein absorption after resistance training.

> In 2012, researchers in the British Journal of Nutrition found that a whey protein dosage of 40g (0.5g/kg of bodyweight) was necessary to maximally stimulate MPS in elderly participants after resistance training.

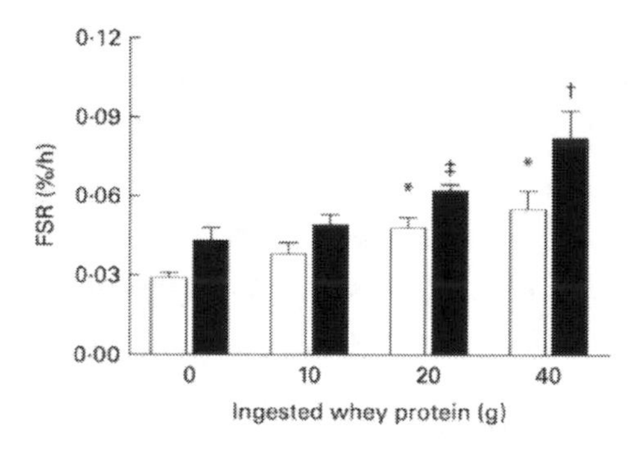

Since the key is getting the amino acids into your bloodstream in and around your workout, you could also try any of the following to help counteract the potential delay in MPS.

- Consume protein shake 'immediately' after your workout.
- Eat a high-protein meal before your workout.
- Sip on half your post-workout protein (or an EAA solution) during your workout.

Other Ways to Get Whey

How you decide to consume whey is up to you, but a protein powder will get you a superior insulin reaction and elevation in muscle protein synthesis (MPS) compared to milk and yogurt. Mainly because powders contain more grams of whey protein per serving, that would be very difficult to obtain by drinking milk (2 cups) or eating yogurt (3 cups). But also because milk and yogurt contain a healthy dose of fat that slows the response.

The other reason whey is preferred is because it doesn't come equipped with a glucose bomb. There's approximately 26g of sugar in 2 cups of 2% milk and 33g of sugar in 3 cups of full-fat yogurt. Go with the skimmed or low-fat options to get the full insulin and MPS effect, and you're looking at 36g in the milk and 57g in the yogurt!

These numbers are especially discouraging for the elderly population, as those with any degree of anabolic resistance would need to consume 3 cups of milk or 4 cups of yogurt to hit 0.5g/kg. Far too much dairy to being consuming in 3 days, let alone after a workout. And a damaging amount for individuals with resistant tissues that will be negatively affected by excess glucose.

Last but not least, is the lactose load in liquid dairy products. Some of the population has gastrointestinal discomfort with a little bit of lactose, and the majority of the population will have gastrointestinal discomfort with the amounts necessary to maximally stimulate MPS. Whey, on the other hand, is virtually lactose-free; and as discussed before, even those that struggle with dairy do just fine with whey protein powder.

What About Raw Dairy?

If you're fortunate enough to live in a country that permits the sale of unpasteurized dairy from grass-fed cattle, this conversation is slightly different. As drinking milk or eating yogurt is a viable option; provided it's understood that you'll need to consume enough to meet the appropriate protein amount (0.3g/kg-0.5g/kg bodyweight).

Fortunately, you can achieve an equivalent insulin reaction to protein powder by adding high-glycemic fruit to your raw dairy. And the difference in MPS is insignificant if you're consuming a high protein meal within a couple hours of your workout.

More importantly, I'd say the MPS is secondary with the additional health benefits you're getting from raw dairy.

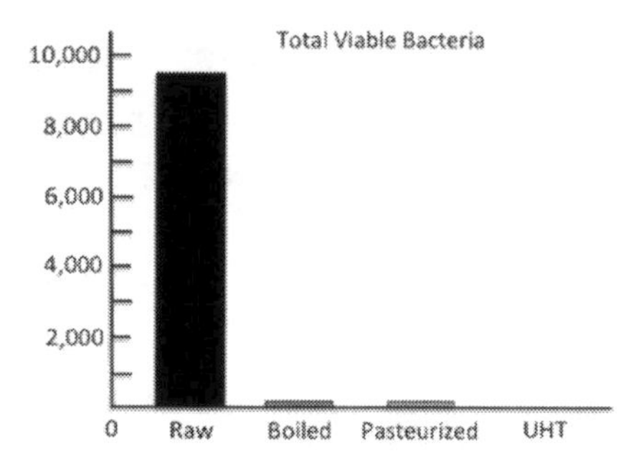

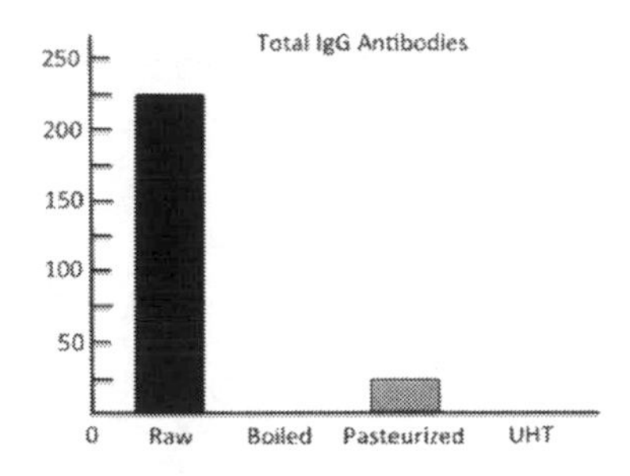

Additionally, raw unpasteurized dairy contains far more whey protein per serving, as heat appears to denature the amount of available protein.

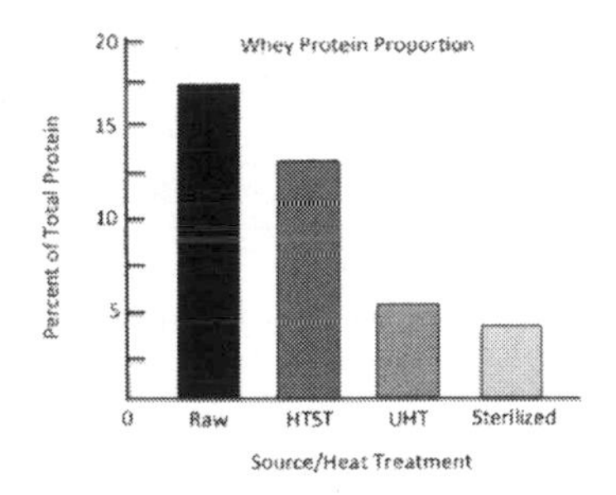

Pasteurized milk can have up to 30% less whey protein compared to raw milk, and 80% less after ultra-high temperature pasteurization

Therefore, raw milk or yogurt is a great alternative to whey protein powder if you can source it. Even though it may not stimulate MPS to the same degree, there comes a point when health and performance collide. One of the reasons we're looking to build muscle is for longevity, and I'd say the beneficial bacteria and antibodies in raw dairy are only promoting that. Plus, it's a higher percentage of whey protein per serving, comes with built-in lactase, and gets you an unmatched level of MPS, without the need to eat excessive amounts of pasteurized milk and yogurt packed with indigestible lactose.

The only thing I'll add with respect to whey protein powders is the convenience factor. Aside from the difficulty obtaining raw dairy, this is one of the reason it's highly encouraged.

Other Ways to Get Leucine

If you've been following along so far, you understand that dairy is superior to animal flesh after exercise because it's rapidly digested. You also recognize that whey protein elevates MPS more than casein, pea, soy, hemp, and rice protein because it's higher in essential amino acids (specifically leucine). Lastly, you accept that the closer whey protein is to its raw natural form the greater the health benefits, while the more it's heated and isolated the greater the MPS response. But what we haven't covered, is why this isolation process isn't taken one step further.

If the essential amino acids are responsible for the rise in MPS, why not separate them entirely and ditch the whey?

Fortunately, this has been done; and you may be more familiar with the resulting product than you think. They're commonly referred to as BCAA's (Branched Chain Amino Acids) or EAA's (Essential Amino Acids) and they come as powdered drink mixes that aim to give you the same MPS benefits of whey, without everything else that comes with it.

In other words, we've taken the isolation of whey 1 step further:

Cow's Milk – Whey Concentrate – Whey Isolate – Whey Hydrolysate – BCAA's

Basically, BCAA's gets rid of any of the side benefits that come with whey protein in an effort to satisfy one goal – elevate MPS.

Research from 2008 in the American Journal of Physiology Endocrinology and Metabolism found a 145% increase in MPS in a group given 20g of 'leucine enriched' EAA's and 30g of carbohydrates 1hr after exercise, compared to 41% in a group given none.

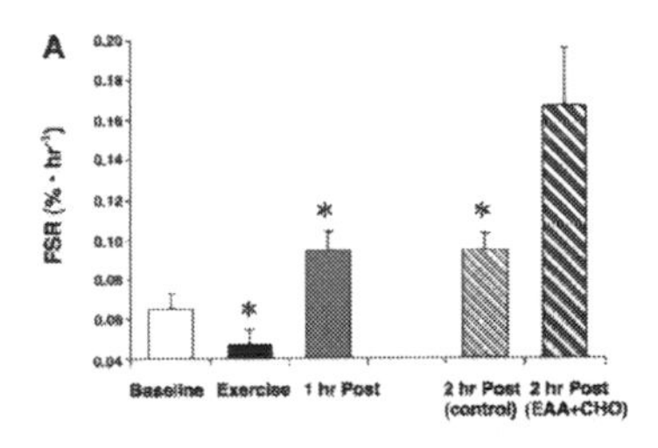

For those with a severe intolerance to whey protein, or extreme discomfort from lactose, this appears to be a viable solution to further elevate MPS after resistance training. But similar to the research on whey protein, an adequate amount of leucine is necessary; and the available evidence suggests that this is approximately 0.03g/kg – 0.05g/kg of bodyweight.

Keeping in mind that those with older muscle, or an insulin resistant body, should look to the upper end of it.

> Research from 2006 in the American Journal of Physiology Endocrinology and Metabolism showed that a 6.7g mixture of EAA's with 26% leucine was not enough to stimulate MPS above baseline in a group of elderly participants, while the same dose with 41% leucine raised MPS to the same level as younger subjects.

Especially for those with, or on the verge of, a certain level of insulin resistance.

Leucine-rich BCAA's appear to be a viable way to spike insulin and MPS and maintain a net positive protein balance after resistance training and before our next meal. For those that can't consume whey, or for times when we can't access whey, this appears to be the next best solution for exploiting the heightened level of MPS after resistance training.

The Perfect POST-Workout Meal

Your post-workout nutrition decision will depend on a variety of individual factors, but I always encourage a high-quality whey isolate because of convenience. Whey is ideal for stimulating muscle growth, as it's rapidly digested and provides the greatest anabolic response. Compared to other proteins, whey also has the highest concentration of leucine, which is essential to stimulating MPS, and promoting the best body composition. Plus, I find it serves as a well-deserved reward for working out.

More than anything we're looking for sustainability, and aside from taking a mini vacation from meat, you'll find that whey serves as a very delicious positive-reinforcer after weight training. Along with enjoying a fruit-smoothie after a job well done, it's the perfect opportunity to mix in some nutrition powerhouses you wouldn't normally eat.

In addition to your whey, water, ice, and carefully selected post-workout fruit (see reference chart in next section), try adding:

- Great Greens – Spinach, Kale, or Swiss Chard
- Super Seeds – Hemp Hearts, Chia Seeds, or Flax Seeds

Sure the fat and fiber might lower the glucose and insulin response, but the benefits you're experiencing from the addition of these foods (anti-inflammatory, feeding gut, etc.) outweighs any negligible reduction.

> A research study from 2004 in the Journal of Applied Physiology found no significant reduction in glycogen content 24 hours after depletion despite adding 165 g fat collectively to the post-exercise recovery meals.

Plus, the breakdown and response from whey is still drastically faster than sitting down to a meal with solid protein and fat.

Whatever you come up with for your post-workout concoction, please make sure it's POST-workout. As just because you have a protein tub in your kitchen, doesn't mean you suddenly turn into a Smoothie Breakfast Barista every morning. Whey still generates a sizeable increase in insulin that is better suited for the post-workout window.

Although some of the literature demonstrates that whey is beneficial as a meal replacement when following a weight-loss strategy, this is generally only seen when replacing carbohydrates. Without resistance exercise, it can help you shed some weight and body fat, but it's not going to do much for lean body mass. And only appears to build muscle when it's concurrent with weight training.

We drink liquid protein AFTER exercise because the insulin secretion is beneficial. It's not beneficial at breakfast, as it will put you in a coma by 10am and have you starting off the day in fat storage mode with a sweet tooth that would get a disciplined man (or woman) in trouble.

> *If you're in a debate between a donut and a whey protein shake, drink the whey; but keep in mind that you're better suited with animal protein.*

Like fruit, whey should be a reward for exercise. This keeps you lean and mean, and leaves you more responsive to the insulin surge after exercise.

Without working out, the only breakfast shake you can get away with is one where the liquid protein is replaced with raw eggs, and the high-glycemic fruit is swapped for berries. Add some great greens, super seeds, and coconut oil, and that's a liquid breakfast we can work with.

To Carb or Not to Carb

With respect to adding carbohydrate to your protein, it all depends on your current body composition. The increased sensitivity of muscle tissue to protein and carbohydrate storage, means we 'should' eat protein and 'can get away' with eating carbohydrates.

It doesn't mean Lean Luke should be ingesting the same amount of carbohydrates as Fat Frank.

Recent evidence has demonstrated that carbohydrate after exercise does not necessarily produce an additive effect on MPS. Likewise, training with low muscle glycogen does not suppress the anabolic response, as researchers once thought it did. The old school thinking that we need to jack up insulin and glucose post-workout to maximize exercise-induced muscular adaptations and facilitate repair of damaged tissue is no more, as we now understand that whey protein, and the essential amino acids that come with it, do a pretty sufficient job at stimulating MPS on their own.

> Research from 2011 in the journal of Medicine & Science in Sports & Exercise looked at consuming 25g of whey protein on it's own, or 25g of whey protein with 50g of added carbohydrates, and aside from a 5-fold higher increase in insulin, MPS and MPB at rest were no different.

For those looking to lose fat, refraining from carbohydrates in the post-exercise period is likely more beneficial, because whey increases fat oxidation.

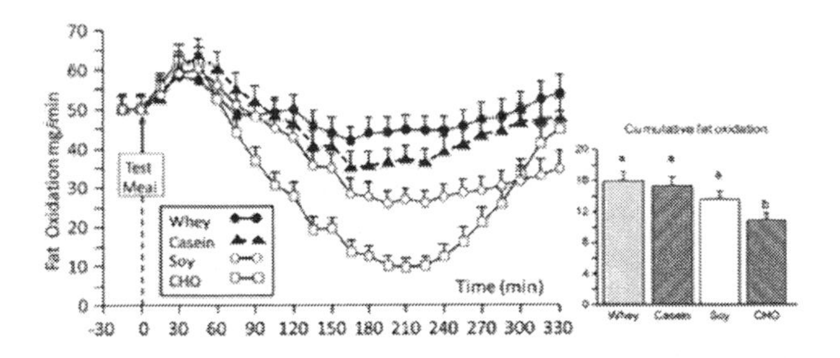

Aside from it's ability to increase energy expenditure, this appears to be driven by the discrepancy created between insulin and glucose levels.

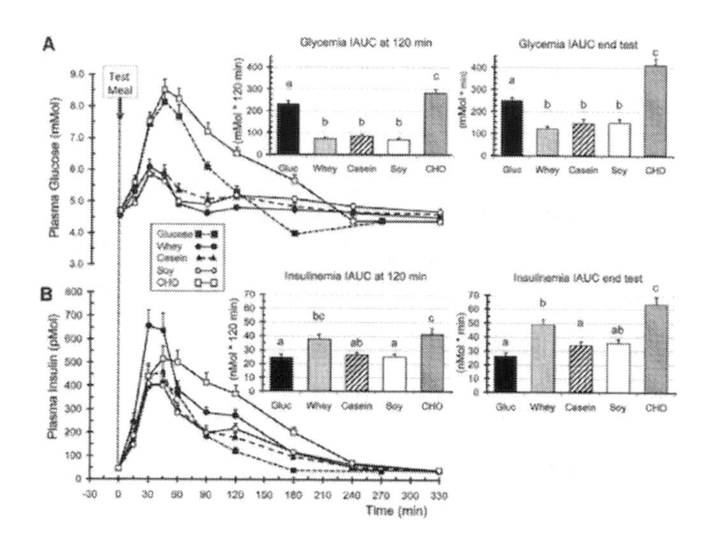

In addition to amino acids stimulating insulin, several of them (leucine, glycine) have the unique ability to lower glucose. This gap creates somewhat of a glucose shortage, which we can either fill with 'good starch,' or leave empty to benefit from increased fat oxidation. Going back to our discussion from *Live It NOT Diet!*, it's best for those with 'lots to lose' to embrace the gap or leave it partially open with lower-glycemic fruit options like berries. Whereas, those with 'visible abs' have the option of rewarding their exercise with higher-glycemic fruit, or waiting until their next solid meal to consume a starchy vegetable, like sweet potatoes.

Here are the reference charts to refresh your memory:

Low-Glycemic		
Berries (All)	Apples	Oranges
Cherries	Peaches/Nectarines	Plums
Watermelon	Cantaloupe	Honeydew Melon
Grapefruit	Pears	Papaya
High-Glycemic		
Banana	Pineapple	Mango
Grapes	Sweet Potato	Taro
Kiwi	Yams	Figs
Very High-Glycemic		
Dried Fruit (All)	Dark Chocolate	100% Fruit Juices
Cassava	White Potato	

Current Body Comp	**Workout Intensity**	**Options**
Lots To Lose	Low	Berries
	High	Berries
Almost There	Low	Low Glycemic Fruit
	High	Low Glycemic Fruit
Lean But No Abs	Low	Low Glycemic Fruit
	High	High Glycemic Fruit or Starch
Visable Abs	Low	High Glycemic Fruit or Starch
	High	2 x High Glycemic or 1 x Very-High Glycemic

**Note: Dried fruits and juices are 'VERY high-glycemic' regardless of type*

For the elderly population that may be experiencing any level of anabolic resistance, sticking to lower-glycemic options is highly encouraged. As extra carbohydrate provides no additional support for MPS, and refraining from excessive glucose will only help improve insulin sensitivity and fat oxidation going forward.

Although some research suggests higher insulin levels equate to less protein breakdown, this is easily achieved with amino acids.

> Evidence from 2008 in the American Journal of Physiology Endocrinology and Metabolism showed that only minimal concentrations of insulin (5mU/L) are required to maximally stimulate protein synthesis, and amounts easily satisfied by whey (30mU/L) necessary to reduce MPB.

In fact, it's been proven that amounts greater than 30mU/L have no further inhibitory effect on muscle breakdown. Suggesting, that any 'extra' is likely unnecessary with respect to insulin and MPS, and amino acids have a large enough impact on insulin to produce a positive change in net protein on their own.

> The administration of insulin in addition to amino acids increases muscle protein synthesis, but this is mainly attributed to the amino acids (hyper aminoacidemia).

It seems the only reason we'd want to add carbohydrate is to further elevate glucose and insulin to replenish glycogen faster. And unless you're training multiple times per day for extended periods of time (cardio) there's not much to replenish. With the high-intensity resistance training we will be performing, you'll be lucky to burn through 20-25% of your muscle glycogen. Equalling approximately 80-100g of glucose, that is replenished pretty quickly with a little bit of fruit.

Realistically, we don't 'need' carbs post-workout to maximize gains in strength and muscle, as the only true benefit from the addition of carbohydrate appears to be glycogen resynthesis. For a lean individual after an intense workout, this may make sense. For an obese, insulin resistant individual with a lot of body fat to lose, it doesn't.

> The leaner you are, and the more intensity you bring to your workout, the more fruit and good starch you can eat AFTER exercise.

We won't necessarily look to increase our carb intake, but rather continue to follow our rule from *Live It NOT Diet!* – "Reward Exercise With Good Starch". The only difference being, you can consume that post-exercise fruit with whey protein.

If you still have a lot to lose, I suggest sticking to the lower glycemic fruits for your treat, as the high insulin and low glucose levels post-workout will help improve your insulin sensitivity over time.

> *Fun Fact: A 2015 study in the International Journal of Molecular Medicine found that consuming ursolic acid (found in apples) with leucine may increase muscle mass more than leucine on it's own.*

How Urgent is Post-Workout Protein?

As demonstrated in a 2012 meta-analysis in the American Journal of Clinical Nutrition, combining protein supplementation with resistance training clearly enhances strength and muscle for participants of all ages and experience levels. What doesn't seem to be clear, is 'when' that protein should be consumed in relation to an exercise session. As some evidence suggests consuming amino acids before is ideal (pre-workout), others say during, (peri-workout) some say immediately after (post-workout), other say before and after, and some say it makes no difference.

So, who do you believe?

Well, fortunately there was a review in 2013 in the Journal of the International Society of Sports Nutrition that analyzed 43 studies to determine the affect of protein timing on muscle and strength gains, and produced results to:

> "refute the commonly held belief that the timing of protein intake in and around a training session is critical to muscular adaptations."

The researchers found that consuming adequate protein in combination with resistance exercise is enough, and there is no significant difference between consuming your protein within 1hr of working out, or greater than 2hrs after.

That being said, what seems to remain constant throughout the available evidence, is that training fasted should be treated differently than training fed. When exercising within a few hours of eating, or immediately after, there's less urgency for post-workout protein because there's already circulating amino acids. But fasted training (ex: first thing in the morning before breakfast, or greater than 3hrs since your last meal), on the other hand, seems to result in a post-workout environment that favors muscle protein breakdown (MPB) if amino acids are not consumed within 60-minutes.

> Research from 2003 in the journal Medicine and Science in Sports and Exercise suggests that MPB is slightly elevated at 60min after resistance training and continues to rise until it results in a negative protein balance at 195min.

If we're thinking realistically, this isn't going to happen. Since no one does heavy resistance training at 6am and avoids eating until 10am. However, it's important to recognize that there's a higher sense of urgency placed on your post-workout protein ingestion if you didn't eat a meal before training. For those with a bit of an odd schedule, this could mean sipping on BCAA's until you're able to sit down for a meal.

With respect to your 'good starch' intake, it appears the timing after resistance training is also somewhat conflicting. Some research discusses a supercompensation effect of glycogen stores immediately after exercise, which can be reduced by 50% if we delay our glucose reload by 2hrs or more. While other evidence seems to suggest that glycogen replenishment 2hrs after exercise is identical to immediate consumption. But after careful review, it seems you should treat your 'good starch' reload the same way you treat your protein:

When training fasted, it's urgent; when training fed, it's not.

I tend to recommend lifting fed later in the day for a variety of reasons (neurological system awake, etc.). However, you need to find the workout and nutrition strategy that works best for you. Because, at the end of the day, that's the one you're going to stick to!

As H. Chtourou and fellow researchers wrote in the Journal of Strength and Conditioning Research in 2012:

> "From a practical point of view, adaptation to strength training is greater at the time of day at which training was scheduled than at other times."

For me, that's training within 1-2hrs of a meal, and consuming my Super Shake anywhere from 30-60 minutes after. If I know I won't be able to have a shake, I will eat a piece of fruit and sip on BCAA's within 30-60 minutes, followed by a meal with lots of protein a few hours later.

As most of my clients can attest to, you'll probably find that your body naturally tells you how urgent the post-workout protein is. If you've had a meal before, you won't be craving it. If you're fasted, it seems you can't consume it quick enough.

"Today's interest in sport is more vicarious than participatory. We idolize the elite athlete who performs for us, rather than the amateur athlete we could and should become."

— Paffenbarger et al, AJE

Go All-Out Occasionally (HIIT it and Quit it)

Believe it or not, you were actually designed to move well. Your body may be preventing you from doing so currently, but that's no indication of what you're capable of. As you learned in Principle #1, shoes, chairs, cars, and computers, have created a restricted, slightly deformed physique that needs to be retrained.

Sadly, this new reality has also made it standard practice to only associate speed, power, and agility with elite athletic performance. Apparently, jumping high and running fast is only for professional athletes, and we're better focusing on improving our cardiorespiratory fitness. Because that's how we stay young and fit right?

Principle #9 is all about getting you to move athletically, by training your speed, power, and agility. We will be adding a 3rd exercise session per week, where you will be taking part in something called high-intensity interval training (HIIT).

HIIT = Brief bouts of all-out exercise (>85%), interspersed with equal (1:1) or longer (1:3) rest periods between sets.

The other option for your 3rd workout of the week, is to add a recreational sport, or higher-intensity activity, like surfing, skiing, or kickboxing. Personally, I get enjoyment out of sprinting, jumping, and throwing around heavy weights, but I understand that this isn't for everyone. Phase 3 is all about adding a 3rd workout to your weekly regimen, where you can push yourself in whatever capacity you're currently at.

That being said, I do hope to see you running fast, jumping high, and being an athlete in the near future. As research suggests that performing these explosive athletic movements in addition to a traditional resistance-training program is critical to increasing the power output that rapidly declines with age.

Go Fast to Burn Fat

Forgetting the fact that a 3rd training sessions per week can increase your results by more than 36%, and all 4 of the high-intensity options we're about to discuss will improve your athletic ability, there's something to be said about the practice of going 'all out.' For instance, research from 2014 in the European Journal of Endocrinology determined that maximal exercise increases a fat burning hormone called irisin (turns white fat to brown) 34% higher than a matched workload with a lower intensity.

Vigorous activity also appears to do a better job activating hormone-sensitive lipase, which is responsible for stimulating fat burning.

> A 2008 study in the International Journal of Obesity researchers compared high-intensity interval (8-sec sprints) and moderate-intensity endurance training over 15 weeks, and despite equal cardiovascular improvements, only saw significant reductions in total fat mass, trunk fat, and fasting insulin levels in the HIIT group.

Even though steady-state aerobic activity may burn more calories and fat during exercise, vigorous activity leads to greater energy expenditure and lipolysis after exercise. Whether this is driven by higher levels of EPOC (excess post exercise oxygen consumption), or fat-burning enzymes and muscle building hormones (gH, testosterone), research has made it quite clear that short-term high-intensity exercise leads to superior reductions in fat loss.

> Research from 2008 in the journal Obesity found significant decreases in total fat mass, visceral belly fat (-9.5%), and fasting insulin (-31%) for a group of women taking part in high-intensity interval exercise, compared to an aerobic group that gained fat mass (0.44kg) and visceral belly fat (10.5%), and experienced far less of a reduction in fasting insulin (9%).

Some have suggested that this increased fat burning is the result of structural and chemical changes to skeletal muscle DNA. These genetic changes (not seen in less intense activity), reprogram the muscle for strength building and fat burning almost immediately. For instance, research in the European Journal of Applied Physiology determined that a 15-min session of HIIT activated 310 genes, compared to only 69 after a 30-minute aerobic session. And more specifically, 16 fat metabolism genes that were active in the HIIT group, were not seen in the steady-state group.

The other likely contributor to this accelerated fat loss is growth hormone (GH). It's also tied to the intensity of exercise, and can increase by nearly 25 times what it is at rest with an all-out intensity.

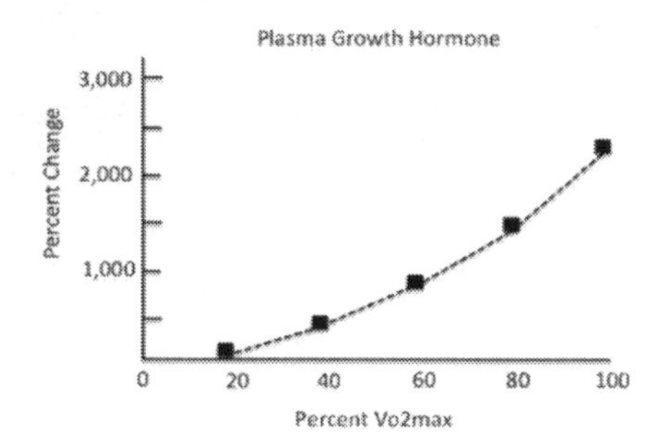

Aside from burning fat and being an anabolic (muscle-burning) hormone on it's own, GH facilitates the increase and uptake of IGF-1 (insulin-like growth factor). Which further stimulates MPS, satellite cells, and receptors that initiate hypertrophy; and is of the reasons low-volume high-intensity exercise preserves muscle, unlike its cardiovascular catabolic cousin.

Go Fast to Last

High-intensity interval exercise also results in far greater improvements in metabolic and cardiovascular health markers compared to moderate-intensity endurance training.

With respect to heart health, research has praised 'low-volume' high-intensity exercise over high-volume moderate-intensity exercise for enhancing vascular structure and function, increasing ventricular mass and stroke volume, improving micro vascular density and enzyme content, controlling blood pressure, and enhancing endothelial function. Despite a MUCH lower training volume and total energy expenditure.

> In 2014, researchers in the journal Menopause, found significant improvements in cardiopulmonary function for a high-intensity exercise group, that were not seen in their continuous training counterparts who exercised twice as long and expended twice the energy.

Endothelial function is arguably the most noteworthy, as it's a precursor for plaque build-up and the development of atherosclerosis. And though exercise in general appears to be a useful intervention for improving it, and preventing the dysfunction that's associated with heart disease, only high-intensity exercise enhances it.

Not surprisingly, it's a similar story with metabolic health. When matched for energy expenditure, 'all out' vigorous physical activity had a greater influence on metabolic syndrome than did moderate intensity physical activity. With various studies demonstrating extremely favorable improvements for vigorous activity in less than 10 minutes of total commitment time.

For instance, researchers in the European Journal of Applied Physiology had individuals take part in 10 min of leisurely bike riding that included only 1-2 short 10-20-sec bursts during the session. After 3 weeks, the participants not only improved their aerobic capacity significantly, but they increased insulin sensitivity by 28%!

This is largely because of HIIT's ability to increase fat burning hormones, while preferentially burning muscle glycogen (stored carbohydrates). Leading to greater fat loss and insulin sensitivity, and superior reductions in fasting glucose and triglycerides.

HIIT is also unique in that it stimulates the fast-twitch muscle fibers that have a considerable impact on delaying the onset of metabolic disease. As discussed, this rapid force production is something that declines with age. And unfortunately it's not always improved with traditional resistance training (in older individuals).

> Bodybuilders that train low intensity and higher rep have smaller type 2 muscle fibers than powerlifters who do high-intensity low reps.

Go Fast to Go Far?

Runner's World and Triathletes will try to tell you otherwise, but HIIT is not only superior in nearly every meaningful health marker, but it provides equivalent improvements in endurance capacity in a fraction of the time.

> In 2010, researchers from the Journal of Physiology found equal aerobic and health improvements from 8-12 sets of 60sec sprints, compared to an endurance-training group exercising almost 98% more.

Despite its inferiority to strength, muscle, metabolic rate, and insulin sensitivity, aerobic capacity (vo2max or peak) remains a valid indicator of total and cardiovascular mortality (whether we have heart disease or not). And aside from aerobic fitness 'burning calories,' this ability to 'improve vo2max' is the other reason it's commonly recommended.

Since we've already discussed the problems with training aerobically, there's no need to go into great detail here. However, I should reiterate that exercising to 'build' strength and muscle, does a pretty spectacular (if not superior) job improving heart health on it's own. Including similar improvements in respiration and aerobic capacity when executed with a high intensity and shorter rest periods.

So, even though we're only lifting weights, we're already increasing our vo2max significantly. That being said, we can improve our vo2max even more by incorporating HIIT. For instance, a study from 2005 in the Journal of Applied Physiology saw participants double their endurance capacity from 26 to 51 minutes in 2 weeks by performing only 6 sessions of 4-7 sprints (30-seconds).

Likewise, researchers in the Journal Physiology compared 90-120min of continuous cycling at 65% intensity, with 4-6 intermittent sprints of 30-seconds and a 4min recovery between sets, to find equal improvements in aerobic capacity.

> Over 2 weeks, the commitment time for the continuous exercise group was 10.5 hours, compared to only 2.5 hours in the HIIT group.

When looking at the difference in power output for HIIT protocols (tall skinny bars), compared to traditional steady-state cardio (solid striped block), I think the ideal training type for building and improving your vo2max is quite obvious:

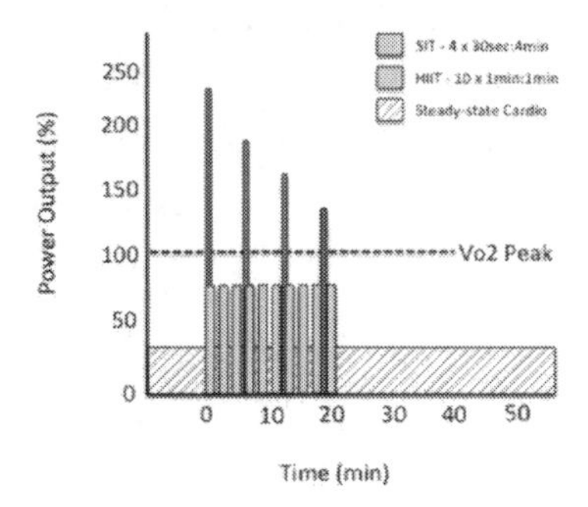

Intensity of exercise has a much bigger impact on Vo2max than duration. And clearly, the more intensity we bring, the greater the improvements.

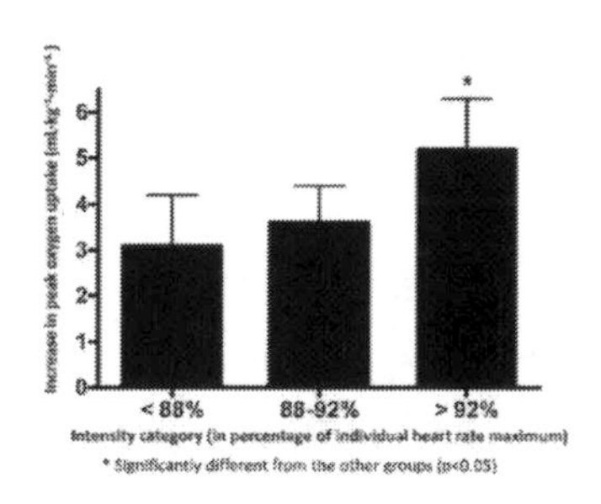

Of interest, the results in the chart above are from a 2014 study in the Journal of Science and Medicine in Sport where researchers tested 112 participants 'with coronary heart disease.' Ultimately, they concluded that:

> "CHD patients who are able to perform high intensity training should aim at increasing exercise intensity above 92% of HR max and thereby possibly achieve even greater improvements in aerobic capacity.

HIIT Improves Anaerobic AND Aerobic Performance

With the efficiency we seek in the rest of our lives, it's quite ironic that steady-state cardio is still as popular as it is. Since a few short bouts of high-intensity exercise increases the body's ability to utilize oxygen, and the capacity for oxidative metabolism in skeletal muscle (the same benefits attributed to endurance training); while improving the 'anaerobic system' simultaneously.

Conversely, aerobic exercise requires far more time and energy, and 'reduces' anaerobic performance. Meaning the more you keep running further and more frequently, the slower you get and less force you generate.

I don't know about you, but I'd rather spend far less time doing the exercise that improves both, as opposed to the one that takes longer and only improves one…?

For all the science geeks out there, HIIT also stimulates markers of AMPK, increases mRNA and genes responsible for energy and metabolic regulation (PGC-1α), and results in greater mitochondrial function and enzyme activity. In other words, any and all of the benefits normally attributed to steady-state aerobic, or continuous moderate-intensity exercise - without the excess time, excess stress, and excess damage that comes with it.

> "The consequences of aerobic exercise are too detrimental to be considered an effective training modality for anaerobic athletes; let alone a necessary one." Charles Pfeiffer, Strength and Conditioning Journal, 2013.

HIIT Options

High Intensity Interval Training (or HIIT) involves performing maximum effort work intervals for short periods of time, followed by equivalent or greater recovery periods. But recently, it was proposed that:

> HIIT be used to describe 'near maximal' intensity of 80-100%, and SIT (sprint interval training) reserved for 'supramaximal' or all out efforts of 100%+.

So, we'll follow a similar guideline with *1% Fitness*, using HIIT to describe our 2-min interval of dynamic exercises, and SIT to identify our 3-min sprint intervals. Generally speaking, sprints are the only activity that give us the ability to truly go 'all out' (at least when compared to jumps, active planks, and step-ups); hence the need for the longer 3-min rest period.

Depending on your experience and comfort level, your execution will fall somewhere along the intensity line of 80-100%+. And being completely frank, most people can't tell the difference between 80 and 90%, so “as fast as you can” seems to be the best approach.

It’s also been proposed that HIIT protocols lasting <10min of total ‘work’ be referred to as ‘low-volume.’ For example, 15 sets of 20-sec sprints would be considered low-volume, because regardless of the rest periods, there’s only 5 minutes of actual work.

With that in mind, the HIIT workouts in *1% Fitness* can all be classified as low-volume.

	Description	**Work (sec)**	**Rest (sec)**	**Sets**
HIIT	Option 1: Leg + Upper/Core	20-30 + 20-30	60-80	10-12
	Option 2: Total Body	20-30	90-100	10-12
SIT	Straight Sprint or All-Out Agility	5-20	160-175	6-8

Level 1 – Low-Impact Bodyweight HIIT

Your introduction to HIIT should be seamless, as Level 1 is very similar in structure to your resistance-training workouts. The only difference between these workouts and your weight-lifting sessions is that the moves are a little more dynamic, and executed with speed. We still want to be under control, but the tempo is more of 1-0-1-0, or even X-0-X-0.

In option 1, you perform a leg exercise for 20-30 seconds, move immediately to an upper body or core exercise for 20-30 seconds, and then rest for the remaining 80 seconds (or whatever's left on the 2-min clock). Similar to your rest option with weight training, you can take a brief rest between the 2 exercises, or move directly to the 2nd movement and rest longer afterwards.

Sample 1 – No rest between
A1 – Box Step-Up – 20 seconds work – 0 seconds rest
A2 – Active Plank – Leg Lifts – 20 seconds work – 80 seconds rest

Sample 2 – 15 sec rest between
A1 – Box Step-Up – 20 seconds work – 15sec rest
A2 – Active Plank – Leg Lifts – 20 seconds work – 65 seconds rest

With option 2, you simply swap the upper-lower superset for a total body movement; like the 'Burpee.' These exercises can be incorporated into the same workout as your upper-lower superset, but they should have their own spot reserved. Experience tells me they're best suited for the END of your workout, but it's your choice.

Sample 1
A1 - Box Step-Up – 20 seconds work – 0 seconds rest
A2 – Active Plank – Leg Lifts – 20 seconds work – 80 seconds rest
B – Burpees – 30 seconds work – 90 seconds rest

Sample 2
A - Burpees – 30 seconds work – 90 seconds rest

B1 - Box Step-Up – 20 seconds work – 0 seconds rest
B2 – Active Plank – Leg Lifts – 20 seconds work – 80 seconds rest

The other option, is to perform all HIIT sets with the same total body exercise. For example, 10 sets of Burpees with a 30sec:90sec work:rest ratio is a great regimen when you're on the road with no access to equipment. I often refer to it "the easiest hardest workout you'll ever do."

Level 2 – High-Impact Bodyweight HIIT

Don't let the name fool you, as these exercises aren't as high impact as you think. The only difference between these HIIT exercises, is that there's a bit more jumping and landing involved. Generally speaking, we want to progressively increase your jumping ability over time, instead of 'jumping' right into it. If you're concerned about your knees, every exercise in the *1% Fitness* plan has an easier alternative that gives you the option to jump less intensely, or not at all.

That being said, jumping may be exactly what your knees need. For instance, research from 2015 in the journal Medicine & Science in Sports & Exercise tested 'progressive' high-impact training on postmenopausal women (50-65 yr old) at risk of osteoporosis and osteoarthritis that were experiencing daily knee pain. Despite a high training frequency of 3 times a week for 12 months, the study found that cartilage quality improved with jumping and rapid agility movements.

It's also what your bones and muscles need, as plyometric training and high power movements are associated with increased bone strength, and fast twitch muscle fiber stimulation.

Level 3 – SIT (Sprint Interval Training

Although sprinting may seem unreachable at the moment, it's an essential component to getting the results you're after. The perfect example is a research study from 2011 in the journal Medicine and Science in Sports and Exercise, where a sprint interval group lost more body fat and experienced equal aerobic improvements with a total training time (with rest) of 6.75 hours, compared to 13.5 hours in the endurance group. The best part being, only 45 minutes of that 6.75 hours was actually spent exercising. Meaning the SIT group spent 5.5% or 1/18th as much time running as the endurance-training group.

The reason sprint intervals are so awesome, is because they permit maximum intensity for the entire body. Allowing us to experience those superior improvements in insulin sensitivity, vo2max, fat loss, fast-twitch fiber recruitment, mitochondrial function, and gene activation.

Before sprint training, make sure you perform the full *1% Fitness* Dynamic Warm-Up, and do a few build-up sprints before your all-out sets. If you're attempting to sprint in barefoot or in your minimalist shoes, performing a few extra foot and ankle drills is also encouraged. As mentioned in Principle #1, we don't want to move right into sprinting barefoot, as your chances of injury are much higher when initially making the switch from shoes. It's extremely important that you work on rebuilding your feet, and feel comfortable walking in minimalist shoes without soreness. We need to thicken the sole of the foot and let the muscles and ligaments properly adapt before attempting barefoot running.

> "While it has been argued that barefoot running may ultimately be less injurious, these data indicate that habitually shod (shoe-wearing) runners who choose to transition into a barefoot technique must undertake the process cautiously." Human Movement Science, 2013

The reasons for going barefoot should be obvious by now, but here are a few additional reasons to make the switch if you're still on the fence:

- *Promotes toe (fore-foot) strike vs. heel (rear-foot) strike in runners* - The reason we rear-foot or heel strike is because our running shoes permit it. The cushioned heel, means we can increase our stride length and drive our heel into the ground with maximum force. Interestingly, even on hard surfaces, barefoot runners generate smaller collision forces than their heel-striking shoe-wearing counterparts. The plantar-flexed foot on landing gives the ankle more give, and decreases the mass delivered to the ground.
- Higher running economy (2-3%) than wearing shoes
- *Less knee stress (patellofemoral joint - 12%) and impact force on the hip* - This is because forefoot landing reduces the impact on the knee, and increases the loading on the Achilles tendon. This is actually a benefit, as the Achilles is designed to absorb more impact stress than the knees. Although, it also serves as a reminder to ease into it!
- Increased running speed (by switching to fore-foot)

During barefoot running, we automatically cushion the foot by plantar-flexing our feet on contact and preventing the shock loading of the limbs that can lead to chronic ailments (shin splints, etc.). We also tend to land mid-foot, which helps build and strengthen the critical muscles and ligaments of the foot

> Research from 1991 in the journal Medicine and Science in Sports and Exercise found that those wearing more expensive running shoes to correct over-pronation or provide more cushioning, experienced more running related injuries.

It's been suggested that footwear is to blame for ankle sprains becoming the most frequently reported acute sports injury. And interestingly, bone and connective tissue injuries related to running are uncommon in developing countries (that don't wear shoes). For example, plantar fasciitis (inflammation of ligament that runs along the sole of the foot) is potentially the most common injury in runners, and it's rarely seen in barefoot populations.

Essentially, shoes give us the ability to be less aware of how we impact the ground. The more the support, the less we moderate.

> "Shoes affect the gait of children. With shoes, children walk faster by taking longer steps with greater ankle and knee motion and increased tibialis anterior activity. Shoes reduce foot motion and increase the support phases of the gait cycle...During running, shoes reduce swing phase leg speed, attenuate some shock and encourage a rear foot strike pattern.." Journal of Foot and Ankle Research, 2011

And it may be even worse with arch supports and orthotics!

I like the way Mark Sisson, the author of *The Primal Blueprint*, puts it when he compares minimalist shoes and traditional shoes to MMA gloves and boxing gloves. The minimalist shoes and MMA gloves have less padding, which means the "I've had enough" message arrives sooner. Conversely, the continuous pounding in heavily cushioned running shoes is like the beating a boxer can take with over-padded gloves.

Any coincidence that boxers are the ones that end up with brain damage?

Level 4 – Weighted HIIT

The most advanced HIIT workout incorporates weighted dynamic movements, like the Kettlebell Swing, Dumbbell Squat and Press, and Med Ball Side Throw. We get to introduce these exercises when we've reached a level of performance that can handle it.

These weighted dynamic maneuvers (like the kettlebell swing) help build explosive muscle and maximal strength even more; and in many cases (like the weighted jump squat) they're more effective at increasing bone density. The nice thing is, the load doesn't have to be substantial. As just like our weight-training workouts, the key is the 'intent' to execute the maneuver with maximal force.

> In a study from 1993 in the journal Medicine & Science in Sports & Exercise, researchers found greater improvement in vertical jump performance from jump squats with a light load (30%) compared to traditional back squats.

Keep in mind, that this doesn't mean we will all of a sudden abandon the bodyweight maneuvers in Level 1 & 2. Instead, we will look to add these weighted options to increase the intensity of our workouts, and get closer to our full athletic potential.

Keeping it Anaerobic – Short Work. Long Rest.

During an initial bout of HIIT training, very little energy is derived from oxidative or aerobic metabolism (requiring oxygen), but this percentage increases with each subsequent set. To avoid turning HIIT training into an aerobic activity, we want to keep our work periods short and our rest periods long.

This smaller work-to-rest ratio also keeps our intensity level as high as possible, since there's less time to push, and more time to recover and restore the short-term energy substrates required to bring maximum intensity to the upcoming set. Specifically, our body has time to clear the build-up of metabolites in muscle tissue (ex: lactate), and our central nervous system has enough time to 'almost' recover completely. I say almost, because there's a strength training phenomenon called the 'post-tetanic potential effect,' which is when your contraction strength is increased after a heavy/explosive set and starts to eventually trickle off. It's been hypothesized that this optimal subsequent set window is around 3-5 minutes.

A short-work and high-rest period is especially important when it comes to sprint interval workouts (SIT), because the maximum intensity is what makes all the difference. For example, research from 2010 in the European Journal of Applied Physiology compared 10-second sprint intervals with 4 minutes rest, to 30-second sprint intervals with 4 minutes rest and found greater peak (96% vs. 89%), average (84% vs. 58%), and minimum power (73% vs. 40%) in the 10-second sprint group. Interestingly, the improvements in Vo2max (9.2% vs. 9.3%) and 30-second sprint performance (8.5% vs. 9.5%) were nearly equivalent, despite double the total work in the 30sec:4min group.

As discussed earlier, the main focus of high-intensity exercise is to stimulate fast-twitch muscle fibers and fat burning, improve insulin sensitivity and mitochondrial function, and potentially enhance our cardiovascular health. Vo2max, oxidative capacity, and the other aerobic performance measures are simply a side effect, and shouldn't become the primary goal of HIIT. Sure they're important predictors of morbidity and mortality, but there's no need to prioritize our training towards improving them. They're secondary to 'going fast,' and they're going to improve regardless of how far (or long) we go.

The perfect example is a training method called 'Tabata,' which consists of 7-8 bouts of 20sec short bursts with 10 seconds of recovery between each set. Despite checking a lot of the boxes for optimal exercise (high-intensity, short duration, total-body movements), and proving extremely useful for improving Vo2peak (15-19% in 4 weeks), the Tabata rest periods are far too short. Essentially, you're looking at one giant set of muscular endurance, that's no different than the 'exhaustive exercise' we discussed earlier.

Don't get me wrong, the odd 5 min bout of all-out effort is encouraged to stress your body in new ways, but there's no reason to perform this style of exercise multiple times per week. Those who do are sacrificing strength, muscle, and power (the most important biomarkers) in favor of endurance (the least).

> Researchers in a 2011 study from the Scandinavian Journal of Medicine and Science in Sports, split participants into a 'resistance training only' group, and 'resistance training plus cardio' group, and found "a clear trend that combined exercise training may impede strength development."

Conversely, when you add short duration high-intensity intervals with plenty of rest to a resistance program, nothing is compromised. Strength is maintained, and both aerobic and anaerobic performance measures improve.

HIIT for Everybody

HIIT is often regarded as an activity for elite athletes only, even though it's proven successful for the very old, very obese, and very sick (diabetes, heart disease). HIIT doesn't require a certain speed, it only asks for your top speed. Which is clearly not as fast as an elite athlete, and obviously not as fast today as it will be. But that's not to say you won't experience the same improvements.

For instance, researchers in the journal Diabetes Care split a group of participants with type 2 diabetes into an 'interval walking' or 'continuous walking' group. The interval walkers alternated every 3 minutes between high-intensity and low-intensity, while the continuous walkers moved at a moderate pace for the full 60 minutes. After performing the protocol 5 days a week for 4 months, the interval group saw a 16-19% increase in Vo2max, compared to no elevation in the continuous group. They also saw significant reductions in fat mass, visceral fat, and fasting glucose, while the continuous group showed no significant improvements in glycemic control.

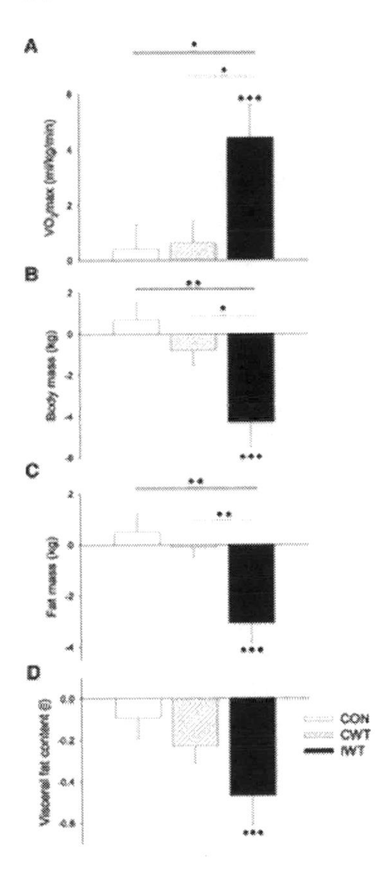

Obviously this is far too much HIIT exercise (5 days/week) to be doing if you're sprinting or doing burpees, but a helpful illustration to show the impact from short bursts of 'intensity' compared to continuous exercise.

HIIT also takes away the two biggest obstacles for not training – time and enjoyment. As a laundry list of research studies report greater enjoyment following HIIT training, when compared to traditional endurance exercise. And adherence is also greater, regardless of current health status (pre-diabetic, diabetic, obese, etc.), or demographic (elderly). Making it the perfect option for those struggling with motivation or scheduling constraints.

> Recent evidence (2015) from the Journal Sports Exercise and Psychology suggests that individuals prefer interval training over continuous, and shorter work intervals (30sec) over longer (120sec).

Aside from the joy of spending a lot less time exercising, this is likely the result of the endorphin spike, that's almost immediate with all out exercise. Compared to endorphin levels that can remain unchanged for hours when the intensity level is below 70%.

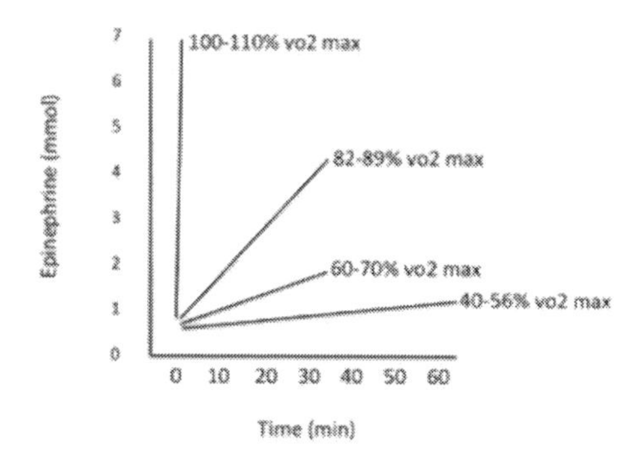

AMPK – The #1 Reason to HIIT it?

AMPK is an energy-regulating enzyme found in the liver, brain, and muscle tissue. When we experience a reduction in available energy, AMPK is stimulated to help ensure there's enough energy molecules to go around.

> When AMPK is elevated, our body flips from storage-mode to burning-mode.

Interestingly, AMPK isn't necessarily stimulated when there's a lack of available 'calories,' but rather a lack of available 'glucose.' Meaning carbohydrate restriction is one of the best ways to stimulate it. As we discussed in *Live It NOT Diet!*, a lack of available glucose makes the body burn fat as fuel (gluconeogenesis). This is partly driven by AMPK, which increases insulin sensitivity (to facilitate glucose uptake) and mitochondrial biogenesis (to manufacture more energy).

The other ways to stimulate AMPK include intermittent fasting, and high-intensity exercise. Again, this is driven by a 'lack of available glucose,' as higher intensity exercise burns mostly glycogen, and AMPK increases as exercise intensity increases.

Fortunately for us, AMPK also has tremendous health benefits. Most of it is aligned with the benefits we've discussed from carbohydrate reduction, but some have referred to AMPK itself as the antithesis of cancer. Mainly because it shuts off cell growth and replication, in order to prioritize burning and breaking down to supply energy.

More specifically, an increase in AMPK appears to block mTOR - a gene that facilitates cancer cell survival and growth. And some evidence suggests that it may actually prevent cancer cells ability to use sugar as fuel.

If that's not enough reason to add an all-out workout to your weekly routine, I don't know what is…?

"The possession of knowledge, unless accompanied by action... is a vain and foolish thing."

—The Kybalion

1% Workouts

Human beings are not designed to 'want' to exercise, we're designed to do what it takes to survive. This is why choosing not to eat when you're hungry, or running for 2hrs is a ridiculous long-term strategy. We already work too much, and relax too little, to be clocking 20miles a week or putting in 90min sessions at the gym every day.

Genetically, we're programmed to move frequently at a slow pace, with infrequent and acute bouts of highly intense movement. When we take part in an exercise regimen that mimics this environment, our body responds with health and performance improvements that can't be matched.

For instance, the chart on the next page shows research results from a study that analyzed the changes in insulin sensitivity using a variety of training methods.

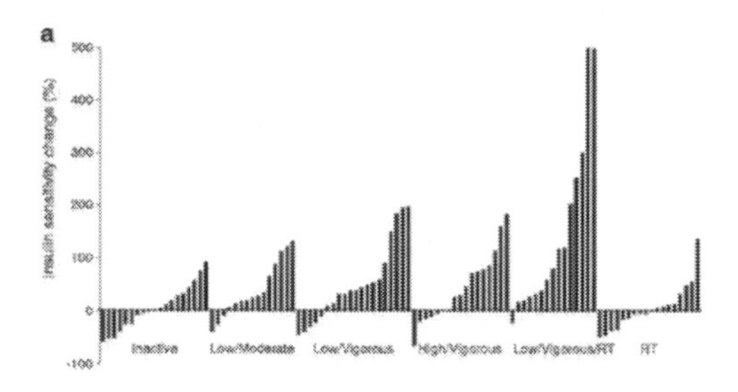

The reason Low-volume Vigorous Activity (HIIT) and Resistance Training produce the best results, is because that's how we're supposed to move!

When we combine a resistance training regimen designed to build strength and muscle, with the cardiovascular and fat burning benefits of HIIT, we create the perfect recipe for a stronger, healthier body. Add the *Live It NOT Diet!* eating strategy, and look to adapt our modern life to mimic our ancestral past, and we're set for a leaner, longer, higher-quality future.

1% Fitness Online

I've done the tedious work of analyzing and reanalyzing the research, and testing and retesting the protocol, and now it's up to you to execute it. The *1% Fitness* workouts are designed to properly progress you from introductory bodyweight movements to advanced resistance-training maneuvers. All exercises should be executed with proper Form and Tempo, and appropriate weight selected to maintain the Rep range and Rest period. If any of these variables can't be met, there needs to be a regression in weight or exercise selection. Luckily, the *1% Fitness* workouts are designed to increase in difficulty from Phase 1 to 3; meaning regressing to an easier exercise choice is as simple as returning to a previously performed variation (ex: bodyweight).

In addition to the workouts posted on the next few pages, please visit:

HTTP://1PERCENTWORKOUTS.COM

There, you can register to access all of the *1% Fitness* workouts online (free of charge), which come equipped with video demonstrations and descriptions of each exercise (by me), and print-ready PDF's to record your weights and track your progress.

This website is also where you'll find the *1% Fitness* Dynamic Warm-up, which should be performed before all Weighted-Resistance and HIIT workouts. Unlike static stretching, which can actually harm your performance (when executed before a workout), a short routine of dynamic activation drills has been shown to enhance strength and power, and may be more effective at preventing injuries. If you'd still like to stretch, it's best executed after strength performance, or in an entirely separate session that won't conflict with a future workout.

Stay Lean (and Good Luck)!

Coach Mike

Mimic Ancestral Movement - Daily

STEP 1: WALK & SQUAT MORE

1. Walk - at least 30-minutes
2. Hold a Deep Squat - 1-3 sets of 30-120sec

STEP 2: SIT & SLOUCH LESS

1. Get Adjustable (sit-to-stand) Workstation – computer at eye level, elbows at or below 90-degrees
2. Take Activity Breaks - 5-10min every 45-60 minutes
3. Stand and Sit Tall – lengthen neck, retract shoulders
4. Counteract Slouching – cat camel, bent-over arm raises, standing scarecrow press, hamstring sweeps, bent-knee leg swings, and the *1% Fitness* Dynamic Warm-Up

STEP 3: UNLEASH YOUR FEET

1. Go Barefoot - when possible
2. Improve Foot Mobility
3. Increase Foot Strength – invisible high-heels, flex-to-point, angled toe points, side rolls, bounce walks, 1-foot balance & grab, sand walking
4. Use Minimalist Shoes

Phase 1 – 2 Weeks (2xWeek)

INSTRUCTIONS

1. Start at Level 1 and work your way up – videos at http://1percentworkouts.com
2. Perform each exercise for 30sec, followed by a 30sec rest (ex: A1 Push-up 30sec, Rest 30sec, A2 Bird Dog 30sec, Rest 30sec, A3…etc.)
3. Don't move to next level until lower level completed with good form for 30sec
4. If can't last 30sec at given level, drop down to lower level to get full 30sec
5. You will likely end up at different levels for different exercises (ex: Bodyweight Squat Level 3, Push-Up Level 1, Glute Bridge Level 2)
6. Do 3 Rounds (Sets) of all Exercises (Ex: A1-A5 3 times through)
7. Total workout time should not exceed 15min - Get a Stopwatch!
8. Perform the workout 2/week with at least 2 days recovery in between
9. If you make it to level 4 there are multiple progressions for some exercises - start at level 1 and only increase with success for 30sec

PHASE 1 – WEEKS 1&2

	Level 1	Level 2	Level 3	Level 4
A1	Push-Up L1	Push-Up L2	Push-Up L3	Push-Up L4
A2	Dead Bug – Bent Knees	Dead Bug – Bent-to-Straight	Dead Bug – Straight Legs	Crossover Crunches (Levels 1-4)
A3	Bodyweight Squat L1	Bodyweight Squat L2	Bodyweight Squat L3	Bodyweight Squat L4
A4	Partial Bird Dog	Full Bird Dog	Standard RKC Plank	Plank Limb Lifts (Levels 1-7)
A5	Glute Bridge L1	Glute Bridge L2	Glute Bridge L4	Glute Bridge L4

**Watch the video demos and record your reps at http://1percentworkouts.com

Phase 2 - 4 Weeks (2xWeek)

PHASE 2.1 – WEEKS 1&2

	Exercise	Tempo	Sets	Reps	Rest
A	Dynamic Warm-Up	1-1-1-1	1	5per	120sec
B1	Front Squat – 1DB Goblet Grip	4-0-1-0	3	10-12	30sec
B2	Seated Overhead Pulldown –Supinated Grip	4-0-1-0	3	10-12	30sec
C1	Straight-Leg Deadlift – Low Pulley Sumo Grip	4-0-1-0	3	10-12	0sec
C2	Seated 45degree Chest Press – 2DB Neutral Grip	4-0-1-0	3	10-12	60sec
D	Standing Pallof Press – Mid Pulley	SLOW	3	10-12 /side	60sec

**Watch the video demos and record your reps and weights at http://1percentworkouts.com

PHASE 2.2 – WEEKS 3&4

	Exercise	Tempo	Sets	Reps	Rest
A	Dynamic Warm-Up	1-1-1-1	1	5per	120sec
B1	Bent-Knee Deadlift – 2DB Suitcase Grip	3-0-1-0	3	6-8	60sec
B2	1-Arm Row From All 4's – 2DB Neutral Grip (Alternating)	3-0-1-0	3	6-8 /side	60sec
C1	Straight-Leg Deadlift) - 1DB Sumo Grip	3-0-1-0	3	6-8	0sec
C2	Flat Chest Press – 2DB Pronated Grip	3-0-1-0	3	6-8	120sec
D	1-Arm Low Farmers Carry – 1DB	SLOW	3	20yds /side	60sec

**Watch the video demos and record your reps and weights at http://1percentworkouts.com

Phase 3 - 8 Weeks (2+1xWeek)

PHASE 3.1 – WEEKS 1&2

	Exercise	Tempo	Sets	Reps	Rest
A	Dynamic Warm-Up	1-1-1-1	1	5per	120sec
B1	Bent-Knee Deadlift – 1DB Sumo Grip	4-0-1-0	3	10-12	30sec
B2	Seated Row –Low Pulley Neutral Grip	4-0-1-0	3	10-12	30sec
C1	1-Arm Standing Overhead Press – 1DB Neutral Grip (Unilateral)	4-0-1-0	3	10-12	30sec
C2	45degree Back Extension – 1DB or Bodyweight	4-0-1-0	3	10-12	30sec
D	High Farmers Carry – 1DB Goblet Grip	SLOW	3	80yds	60sec

PHASE 3.1 - HIIT

	Exercise	Sets	Work	Rest
A	Dynamic Warm-Up	1	5per	120sec
B1	Step-Up + Knee Drive	3	20sec	20sec
B2	Active Plank - Foot Walks	3	20sec	60sec
C1	Sumo Squat + Kick/Knee Drive	3	20sec	20sec
C2	Active Plank - Tricep Get Ups	3	20sec	60sec

**Watch the video demos and record your weights/reps at http://1percentworkouts.com

PHASE 3.2 – WEEKS 3&4

	Exercise	Tempo	Sets	Reps	Rest
A	Dynamic Warm-Up	1-1-1-1	1	5per	120sec
B1	Straight-Leg Deadlift (Hip Hinge) – 2DB Suitcase Grip	3-0-1-0	3	6-8	60sec
B2	Flat Chest Press – 2DB Half Twisting Grip (Neutral-to-Pronated)	3-0-1-0	3	6-8	60sec
C1	Inverted Row – Supinated Grip (Incline or Flat)	3-0-1-0	3	6-8	0sec
C2	Standard Lunge – 2DB Front Foot Elevated (Unilateral)	3-0-1-0	3	6-8 /side	120sec
D	45degree Iso Hold – Bodyweight (L1-3)	HOLD	3	30sec /side	60sec

PHASE 3.2 - HIIT

	Exercise	Sets	Work	Rest
A	Dynamic Warm-Up	1	5per	120sec
B1	Speed Skaters or Sprinter Starts	4	20sec	10sec
B2	V-Ups (L1-4)	4	20sec	70sec
C	Elevated Burpee + Step or Jump up	4	30sec	90sec

**Watch the video demos and record your weights/reps at http://1percentworkouts.com

PHASE 3.3 – WEEKS 5&6

	Exercise	Tempo	Sets	Reps	Rest
A	Dynamic Warm-Up	1-1-1-1	1	5per	120sec
B1	Front Squat - 2DB Neutral Grip	4-0-1-0	4	8-10	30sec
B2	15degre Prone Row – 2DB Neutral Grip	4-0-1-0	4	8-10	30sec
C1	Seated Overhead Press (Unsupported) – 2DB Pronated Grip	4-0-1-0	4	8-10	0sec
C2	Glute Bridge – 1DB Back on Bench	4-0-1-0	4	8-10	60sec
D	Hanging Iso-Hold – Knee's at 90	HOLD	3	30sec	60sec

PHASE 3.3 - SIT

	Exercise	Sets	Work	Rest
A	Dynamic Warm-Up	1	5per	120sec
B	Build-Up Sprints – 40-90%	4	30sec	130sec
C	All-Out Sprints (90-110%)	6	15sec	165sec

**Watch the video demos and record your weights/reps at http://1percentworkouts.com

PHASE 3.4 – WEEKS 7&8

	Exercise	Tempo	Sets	Reps	Rest
A	Dynamic Warm-Up	1-1-1-1	1	5per	120sec
B1	Bent-Knee Deadlift (to Rack/Step) – BB Standard Grip	3-0-1-0	4	4-6	30sec
B2	45degree Chest Press – BB Standard Grip	3-0-1-0	4	4-6	90sec
C1	Assisted Pull-Up - Neutral Grip	3-0-1-0	4	4-6	60sec
C2	Standard Split-Squat – 2DB Front Foot Elevated or Flat (Unilateral)	3-0-1-0	4	4-6 /side	60sec
D	1-Arm Overhead Farmers Carry – 1DB	SLOW	3	40yds /side	60sec

PHASE 3.4 - HIIT

	Exercise	Sets	Work	Rest
A	Dynamic Warm-Up	1	5per	120sec
B1	Sumo Deadlift + Overhead Press – 1DB or Med Ball	3	20sec	10sec
B2	Active Plank – 1DB Pull Across	3	20sec	70sec
C1	Skier on Step or Standard Step-Ups	3	20sec	10sec
C2	V-sit + Med Ball Hold or Press	3	20sec	70sec

**Watch the video demos and record your weights/reps at http://1percentworkouts.com

About The Author

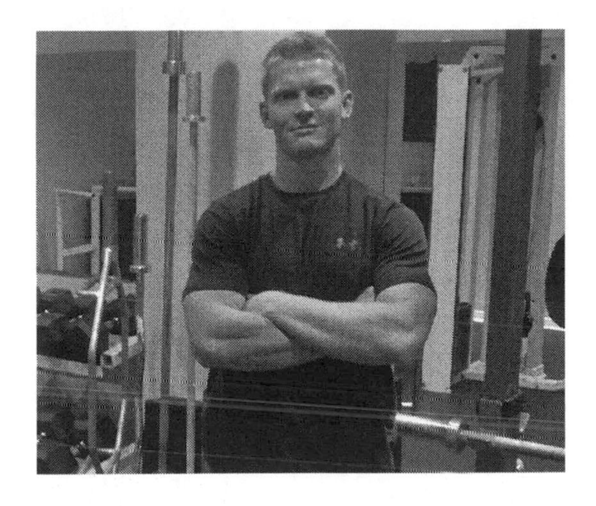

Mike Sheridan has been advising on nutrition and fitness for nearly a decade. His success is due in large part to his philosophy, that 'Transformation Starts With Education.' Not just showing his clients what to do, but teaching them why.

In addition to his 3-Step Transformation Plan (*Eat Meat And Stop Jogging, Live It NOT Diet!, and 1% Fitness*), 'Coach' Mike continues to share his knowledge and experience via guest articles, blog posts, and personal appearances.

References

Introduction

Booth FW, et al. 1993. Structural aspects of aging human skeletal muscle. In Musculoskeletal Soft Tissue Aging Impact on Motility, ed. Rosemont, IL: American Academy of Orthopaedic Surgeons.

Rosenberg IH. 1997. Sarcopenia: Origins and clinical relevance. J Nutr 127(5):9905-9915.

Fielding RA, et al. 2015. Emerging Impact of Skeletal Muscle in Health and Disease. Calc Tiss Inter 96(3):181-182.

Fielding RA, et al. 2011. Sarcopenia: an undiagnosed condition in older adults. Current consensus definition: prevalence, etiology, and consequences. International working group on sarcopenia. J Am Med Dir Assoc 12:249–256.

Akasaki Y, et al. 2014. Glycolytic fast-twich muscle fiber restoration counters adverse age-related changes in body composition and metabolism. Aging Cell 13(1):80-91.

Stenholm S, et al. 2014. Obesity and muscle strength as long-term determinants of all-cause mortality – a 33-year follow-up of the Mini-Finland Health Examination Survey. Int J Obes (Lond) 38(8):1126-32.

Ling CH, et al. 2010. Handgrip strength and mortality in the oldest old population: the Leiden 85-plus study. CMAJ 182(5):429-35.

Puthucheary ZA, et al. 2013. Acute skeletal muscle wasting in critical illness. JAMA 310:1591–1600.

Bauer J, et al. 2013. Evidence-based recommendations for optimal dietary protein intake in older people: a position paper from the PROT-AGE Study Group. J Am Med Dir Assoc 14:542–559.

Warden SJ, et al. 2014. Physical activity completed when young has residual bone benefits at 94 years of age: a within-subject controlled case study. J Musculoskelet Neuronal Interact 14(2):239-43.

Shaw KA, et al. 2006. Exercise for overweight or obesity (Review). Cochrane Database of Systematic Reviews 4:CD003817.

Finlayson G, et al. 2009. Acute compensatory eating following exercise is associated with implicit hedonic wanting for food. Physiol Behav 97(1):62-7.

Turner JE, et al. 2010. Nonprescribed physical activity energy expenditure is maintained with structured exercise and implicates a compensatory increase in energy intake. Am J Clin Nutr.

Manthou E, et al. 2010. Behavioural compensatory adjustments to exercise training in overweight women. Med Sci Sport Exer 42(6):1121-1128.

Graf CE, et al. 2015. Body composition and all-cause mortality in subjects older than 65y. Am J Clin Nutr 101(4):760-767.

Garrow JS, et al. 1995. Meta-analysis: effect of exercise, with or without dieting, on the body composition of overweight subjects. Eur J Clin Nutr 49:1–10.

Sartor F, et al. 2010. High-intensity exercise and carbohydrate-reduced energy-restricted diet in obese individuals. Eur J Appl Physiol 110(5):893-903.

Principle #1

Shaw, Colin. "How Far Fitness Has Fallen." Outside Online. 26 Apr. 2014. <http://www.outsideonline.com/fitness/bodywork/the-fit-list/How-Far-Fitness-Has-Fallen.html>.

O'Keefe J, et al. 2011. Exercise Like a Hunter-Gatherer: A Prescription for Organic Physical Fitness. Progress in Cardiovascular Disease. 53(6), 471-479.

Troiano RP, et al. 2008. Physical activity in the United States measured by accelerometer. Med Sci Sport Exer 40(1):181-188.

Health and Social Care Information Centre. 2009. Health Survey for England—2008: Physical Activity and Fitness http://www.hscic.gov.uk/pubs/hse08physicalactivity

Colley RC, et al. 2011. Physical activity of canadian children and youth: accelerometer results from the 2007 to 2009 canadian health measures survey. Health Reports 22 (1):15-23.

Bassett DR, et al. 2010. Pedometer-measured physical activity and health behaviors in U.S. adults. Med Sci Sport Exer 42(10)1819-1825.

Aoyagi Y, et al. 2010. Habitual physical activity and health in the elderly: the Nakanojo study. Geriatrics Gerontology International 10(1):S236–43.

Miyahita M, et al. 2008. Accumulating short bouts of brisk walking reduces postprandial plasma triacylglycerol concentrations and resting blood pressure in healthy young me. Am J Clin Nutri 88(5):1225-1231.

van Uffelen JGZ, et al. 2007. Walking or vitamin B for cognition in older adults with mild cognitive impairment? A randomized controlled trial. Br J Sports Med.

Vreugdenhil A, et al. 2012. A community-based exercise programme to improve functional ability in people with Alzheimer's disease: a randomized controlled trial. Scan J Caring Sci 26(1):12-9.

Pollock ML, et al.1991. Injuries and adherence to walk/jog and resistance programs in elderly. Med Sci Sport Exerc 23:1194-1200.

Terjung, R. 1979. Endocrine response to exercise. Exerc Sport Sci Rev 7:153-79. New York: MacMillan.

Miyatake N, et al. 2002. Daily walking reduces visceral adipose tissue areas and improves insulin resistance in Japane obese subjects. Diab Res Clin Prac 58(20):101-107.

Mikus C, et al. 2012. Lowering Physical Activity Impairs Glycemic Control in Healthy Volunteers. Med Sci Sport Exerc 2012. 44(2), 225-231.

Brooks G, et al. 1994. Balance of carbohydrate and lipid utilization during exercise: The "crossover" concept. J Appl Physiol 76:2253-61.

Goto K, et al. 2007. Enhancement of fat metabolism by repeated bouts of moderate endurance exercise. J App Physiol 102(6):2158-2164.

Mathur N, et al. 2008. Exercise as a means to control low-grade systemic inflammation. Media Inflam 109502.

Sun Q, et al. 2010. Physical activity at midlife in relation to successful survival in women at age 70 years or older. Arch Intern Med 170(2):194-201.

Hayashi T, et al. 1999. Walking to work and the risk of hypertension in men: The Osaka Health Survey. Ann Intern Med 131(1):21-26.

Lautenschlager NT, et al. 2008. "Effect of Physical Activity on Cognitive Function in Older Adults at Risk for Alzheimer Disease: A Randomized Trial." JAMA 300(9):1027-37.

Schaefer S, et al. 2010. Cognitive performance is improved while walking: Differences in cognitive-sensorimotor couplings between children and young adults. Eur J Dev Psy 7(3):371-389.

Laurin D, et al. 2001. Physical activity and risk of cognitive impairment and dementia in elderly persons. Archives Neurology 58:498-504.

Ravaglia G, et al. 2008. Physical activity and dementia risk in the elderly. Neurology 70(19 Pt 2):1786-1794.

Bartholomew JB, et al. 2005. Effects of acute exercise on mood and well-being in patients with major depressive disorder. Med Sci Sport Exer 37(12):2032-2037.

Buchman AS, et al. 2012. Total Daily Physical Activity and the Risk of AD and Cognitive Decline in Older Adults. Neurology 78(17):1323-29.

Weuve J, et al. 2004. Physical Activity, Including Waking, and Cognitive Function in Older Women. JAMA 292(12):1454-61.

Ownby RL, 2006. Medication adherence and cognition medical, personal and economic factors influence level of adherence in older adults. Geriatrics 61(2):30–5.

Strandberg TE, et al. 2009. Predictors of mortality in home-dwelling patients with cardiovascular disease aged 75 and older. J Amer Geriat Soc 57(2):279–84.

Yavari A, et al. 2010. The Effect of Aerobic Exercise on Glycosylated Hemoglobin Values in Type 2 Diabetes Patients. Journal of Sports Medicine and Physical Fitness 50(4):501-05.

Crane PK, et al. 2013. Glucose levels and risk of dementia. N Engl J Med 369:540-548.

Carson AP, et al. 2014. Hemoglobin A1c and the progression of coronary artery classification among adults without diabetes. Diabetes Care.

Knowler WC, et al. 2002. Reduction in the incidence of type 2 diabetes with lifestyle intervention or metformin," N Engl J Med 346(6):393-403.

Saydah SH, et al. 2002. Abnormal glucose tolerance and the risk of death in the United States. Am J Epidemiol 157(12):1092-1100.

Hildebrand JS, et al. 2013. Recreational Physical Activity and Leisure-Time Sitting in Relation to Postmenopausal Breast Cancer Risk. Cancer Epidemiol Biomarkers Prev 22 (10):1906-12.

Myers J. 2003. Exercise and Cardiovascular Health. Circulation 107:e2-e5.

Brownson RC, et al. 2005. Declining rates of physical activity in the United States: what are the contributors? Annu Rev Public Health 26:421–43.

American Psychological Association. "Sedentary Lives Can Be Deadly: Physical Inactivity Poses Greatest Health Risk To Americans, Expert Says." ScienceDaily. ScienceDaily, 10 August 2009. <www.sciencedaily.com/releases/2009/08/090810024825.htm>.

Wilmot EG, et al. 2013. Sedentary time in adults and the association with diabetes, cardiovascular disease and death: a systematic review and meta-analysis. Diabetologia 55(11):2895-905.

Biswas A, et al. 2015. Sedentary time and its association with risk for disease incidence, mortality, and hospitalization in adults: a systematic review and meta-analysis. Ann Intern Med 162(2):123-132.

George ES, et al. 2013. Chronic disease and sitting time in middle-aged Australian males: findings from the 45 and Up Study. Inter J Behav Nutr Phys Activ 10:20.

Matthews CE, et al. 2012. Amount of time spent in sedentary behaviors and cause-specific mortality in US adults. Am J Clin Nutr 95:437–45.

Schmid D, et al. 2014. Sedentary behavior increases the risk of certain cancers. JNCI J Natl Cancer Inst 106(7):dju206.

George SM, et al. 2010. Beyond recreational physical activity: examining occupational and household activity, transportation activity, and sedentary behavior in relation to postmenopausal breast cancer risk. Am J Public Health 100:2288–95.

Kruk J. 2009. Lifetime occupational physical activity and the risk of breast cancer: a case-control study. Asian Pac J Cancer Prev 10:443–8

O'Neill, R. "Standing - Hazards Magazine." Standing - Hazards Magazine. 1 Aug. 2005. <http://www.hazards.org/standing/index.htm>.

Chaput JP, et al. 2015. Workplace standing time and the incidence of obesity and type 2 diabetes: a longitudinal study in adults. BMC Public Health 15:111.

Saunders TJ, et al. 2013. Sedentary behaviour, visceral fat accumulation and cardiometabolic risk in adults: a 6-year longitudinal study from the Quebec Family Study. PLoS One 8(1):e54225.

Tudor-Locke C, et al. 2004. How many steps/day are enough? Preliminary pedometer indices for public health. Sports Med 34(1):1-8.
Healy GN, et al. 2008. Breaks in sedentary time: beneficial associations with metabolic risk. Diabetes Care 31:661–6.

Healy GN, 2011. Sedentary time and cardio-metabolic biomarkers in US adults: NHANES 2003- 06. Eur Heart J 32:590–7.

Peddie MC, et al. 2013. Breaking prolonged sitting reduces postprandial glycemia in healthy, normal-weight adults: a randomized crossover trial. Am J Clin Nutr 98(2):358-366.

Srinivasan B, et al. 2015. Light-Intensity Physical Activities and Mortality in the United States General Population and CKD Subpopulation. CJASN.

May S, et al. 2011. High frequency of McKenzie's postural syndrome in young population of non-care seeking individuals. J Man Manip Ther 19(1):48-54.

Mörl F, et al. 2013. Bradl I. Lumbar posture and muscular activity while sitting during office work. J Electromyogr Kinesiol 23(2):362-8.

McGill, SM. "The Painful Lumbar Spine." Www.ideafit.com. 1 Jan. 2010. <http://www.ideafit.com/fitness-library/the-painful-lumbar-spine>.

Thompson JA, et al. 2013. Gluteus maximus and soleus compensate for simulated quadriceps atrophy and activation failure during walking. J Biomech 46(13):2165-72.

Hossain M, et al. 2005. A model of dynamic sacro-iliac joint inability from malrecruitment of gluteus maximus and biceps femoris muscles resulting in low back pain. Med Hypotheses 65(2):278-81.

Lewis CL, et al. 2007. Anterior hip joint force increases with hip extension, decreased gluteal force, or decreased iliopsoas force. J Biomech 40(16):3725-31.

Barker PJ, et al. 2013. Anatomy and biomechanics of gluteus maximus and the thoracolumbar fascia at the sacroiliac joint. Clin Anat.

Sikirov D. 2003. Comparison of straining during defecation in three positions: results and implications for human health. Dig Dis Sci 48(7):1201–5.

Mulholland SJ, et al. 2001. Activities of daily living in non-Western cultures: range of motion requirements for hip and knee joint implants. Int J Rehabil Res 24(3):191-8.

Hemmerich A, et al. 2006. Hip, knee, and ankle kinematics of high range of motion activities of daily living. J Orthop Res 24(4):770-81.

Salem G, et al. 2001. Patellofemoral joint kinetics during squatting in collegiate women athletes. Clin Biomech (Briston, Avon) 16(5):424-30.

Klein K. 1961. The deep squat exercise as utilized in weight training for athletes and its effects on the ligaments of the knee. J Assoc Phys Ment Rehabil 15:6–11.

Klein K. 1962. The knee and the ligaments. J Bone Joint Surg 44-A:1191–1193.

Underwood J. 1962. The knee is not for bending. Sports Illustrated 16:50.

Meyers E. 1971. Effect of selected exercise variables on ligament stability and flexibility of the knee. Res Q 42: 411–422.

Li G, et al. 1999. The importance of quadriceps and hamstring muscle loading on knee kinematics and in-situ forces in the ACL. J Biomech 32:395–400.

Kanamori A, et al. 2000. The forces in the anterior cruciate ligament and knee kinematics during a simulated pivot shift test: A human cadaveric study using robotic technology. Arthroscopy 16:633–639.

Sakane M, et al. 1997. In situ forces in the anterior cruciate ligament and its bundles in response to anterior tibial loads. J Orthop Res 15:285–293.

Markolf KL, et al. 1996. Effects of combined knee loadings on posterior cruciate ligament force generation. J Orthop Res 14:633–638.

Lorenzetti S, et al. 2012. Comparison of the Angles and Corresponding Moment in the Knee and Hip during Restricted and Unrestricted Squats. J Strength Cond Res.

Li G, et al. 2004. In situ forces of the anterior and posterior cruciate ligaments in high knee flexion: An in vitro investigation. J Orthop Res 22:293–297.

Schoenfeld BJ. 2010. Squatting kinematics and kinetics and their application to exercise performance. J Strength Cond Res. 24(12):3497-506.

Lamontagne M, et al. 2009. The effect of cam FAI on hip and pelvic motion during maximum squat. Clin Orthop Relat Res. 467(3):645-50.

Weiss L, et al. 2000. Comparative effects of deep versus shallow squat and leg-press training on vertical - jumping ability and related factors. J Strength Cond Res 14:241–247.

Caterisano A, et al. 2002. The effect of back squat depth on the EMG activity of 4 superficial hip and thigh muscles. J Strength Cond Res 16: 428–432.

Bloomquist K, et al. 2013. Effect of range of motion in heavy load squatting on muscle and tendon adaptations. Eur J Appl Physiol.

Esformes JI, et al. 2013. Effect of back squat depth on lower body post-activation potentiation. J Strength Cond Res.

Hartmann H, et al. 2012. Influence of squatting depth on jumping performance. J Strength Cond Res 26(12):3243-61.

Matuschek C, et al. 2012. Influence of Squatting depth on Jumping Performance. J Strength Cond Res 26(12):3243-3261.

Universiteit Antwerpen. "Footwear Alters Normal Form And Function Of The Foot." ScienceDaily. ScienceDaily, 24 July 2009. <www.sciencedaily.com/releases/2009/07/090724091339.htm>.

Robbins SE, et al. 1987. Running-related injury prevention through barefoot adaptations. Med Sci Sport Exerc 19:148-156.

Frederick EC. 1986. Kinematically mediated effects of sports shoe design: a review. J Sport Sci 4:169-184.

Wegener C, et al. 2011. Effect of children shoes on gait: a systematic review and meta-analysis. J Foot Ankle Res 4:3.

Sachithanandam V, et al. 1995. The influence of footwear on the prevalence of flat foot: a survey of 1846 skeletally mature persons. J Bone Joint Surg 77-B:254-7.

Yessis M. 2000. Explosive running. Illinois, USA. Contemporary Books.

Robbins S, et al. 1993. Protective sensation of the plantar aspect of the foot. Foot and Ankle 14, 347-352.

Principle #2

Roth SM, et al. 2000. Strength training for the prevention and treatment of sarcopenia: sarcopenia in aging. J Nutr Health Aging. 2000;4(3):143–155.

Vincent G. and Velkoff V. 2013. In: The Next Four Decades: The Older Population in the United States 2010 to 2050. US Department of Commerce EaSA, editor. pp. 25–1138.

Lexell J, et al. 1987. What is the cause of the ageing atrophy? J Neur Sci 84(2-3):275-294.

Evans W. and Rosenberg I. (1991) Biomarkers. Simon & Schuster, New York, NY.

Evans WJ. 1998. Exercise and nutritional needs of elderly people: effects on muscle and bone. Gerodontology 15(1):15–24.

Guralnik JM, et al. 1993. Physical disability in older Americans. J Gerontol. 48(Spec No):3–10.

Sayer AA, et al. 2007. Grip strength and the metabolic syndrome: findings from the Hert-fordshire Cohort Study. QJM 100: 707.

Hunter GR, et al. 1997. Fat distribution, physical activity, and cardiovascular risk factors. Med Sci Sports Exerc 29: 362-9.

Williams MJ, et al. 1997. Regional fat distribution in women and risk of cardiovascular disease. Am J Clin Nutr 65: 855-60.

Cherbuin N, et al. 2012. Higher normal fasting plasma glucose is associated with hippocampal atrophy: The Path Study. Neurology 79(10):1019-1026.

Macaluso A, et al. 2004. Muscle strength, power and adaptations to resistance training in older peole. Eur J Appl Physiol 92(4):450-72.

Short K. et al. 2005. Changes in myosin heavy chain mRNA and protein expression in human skeletal muscle with age and endurance training. J App Physiol 99:95-102.

Pette D. 2001. Historical Perspectives: Plasticity of mammalian muscle. J App Physiol 90(3):1119-24.

Hunter GR, et al. 2004. Effects of resistance training on older adults. Sports Med 34 (5):329-48.

Hurley BF, et al. 2000. Strength training in the elderly: effects on risk factors for age-related diseases. Sports Med 30:249-68.

Nelson ME, et al. 1994. Effects of high-intensity strength training on multiple risk factors for osteoporotic fractures: a randomized controlled trial. JAMA 272:1909-14.

Fiatarone MA, et al. 1994. Exercise training and nutritional supplementation for physical frailty in very elderly people. N Engl J Med 330(25):1769–1775.

Latham NK, et al. 2004. Systematic review of progressive resistance strength training in older adults. J Gerontol A Biol Sci Med Sci. 59(1):48–61.

Miller JP, et al. 1994. Strength training increases insulin action in healthy 50-to 65-year-old men. J Appl Physiol 77: 1122-7.

Prately R, et al. 1994. Strength training increases resting metabolic rate and norepinephrine levels in healthy 50- to 65-yr-old men. J Appl Physiol 76:133-7.

Fleck SJ. 1988. Cardiovascular adaptations to resistance training. Med Sci Sports Exerc. 20:S146-51.

Porter C, et al. 2014. Resistance exercise training alters mitochondrial function in Human Skeletal Muscle. Med Sci Sports Exerc.

Cauza E, et al. 2005. The relative benefits of endurance and strength training on the metabolic factors and muscle function of people with type 2 diabetes mellitus. Arch Phys Med Rehabil 86:1527-1533.

Baar K. 2006. Training for endurance and strength: lessons from cell signaling. Med. Sci. Sports Exerc. 38:1939-1944.

Anderson T, et al. 1982. Effects of three resistance training programs on muscular strength and absolute and relative endurance. Res Q 53:1-7.

Mekary RA, et al. 2015. Weight training, aerobic physical activities, and long-term waist circumference change in men. Obesity 23(2):461-7.

Balducci S, et al. 2004. Is a long term aerobic plus resistance training program feasible for and effective on metabolic profile in type 2 diabetes? Diabetes Care 27: 841-2.

Castaneda C, et al. 2002. A randomized controlled trial of resistance exercise training to improve glycemic control in older patients with type 2 diabetes. Diabetes Care 25:2335-41.

Dunstan DW, et al. 2002. High-intensity resistance training improves glycemic control in older patients with type 2 diabetes. Diabetes Care 25:1729-36.

Hunter GR, et al. 2000. Resistance training increases total energy expenditure and free-living physical activity in older adults. J Appl Physiol 89:977-84.

Hunter GR, et al. 2002. Resistance training and intra-abdominal adipose tissue in older men and women. Med Sci Sports Exerc 34:1023-28.

Schmitz KH, et al. 2003. Strength training for obesity prevention in midlife women. Int J Obes Relat Metab Disord 27:326-33.

Treuth MS, et al. 1994. Effects of strength training on total and regional body composition in older men. J Appl Physiol 77:614-20.

Treuth MS, et al. 1995. Reduction in intra-abdominal adipose tissue after strength training in older women. J Appl Physiol 78:1425-31.

Wolfe RR. 2006. The underappreciated role of muscle in health and disease. Am J Clin Nutr 84:475-82.

Weinsier RL, et al. 2002. Free-living activity energy expenditure in women successful and un- successful in maintaining a normal body weight. Am J Clin Nutr 75:499-504.

Campbell WW, et al. 1994. Increased energy requirements and changes in body composition with resistance training in older adults. Am J Clin Nutr 60:167-75.

Treuth MS, et al. 1995. Energy expenditure and substrate utilization in older women after strength training: 24 hour metabolic chamber. J Appl Physiol 78:2140-6.

Milesky A, et al. 1991. Changes in muscle fiber size and composition in response to heavy resistance exercise. Med Sci Sports Exerc 23:1042-49.

MacDougall J. 1992. Hypertrophy or Hyperplasia. In Strength and Power in Sport, ed 230-38. London: Blackwell Scientific Publishing.

Brown AB, et al. 1990. Positive adaptations to weight-lifting training in the elderly. J Appl Physiol 69(5):1725–1733.

Goldberg AP. 1989. Aerobic and resistance exercise modify risk factors for coronary heart disease. Med Sci Sports Exerc 21:669-74.

Hurley BF, et al. 1987. Effects of weight training on risk factors for coronary heart disease. Sports Med 4:231-8.

Roberts CK. 2013. Untrained young men have dysfunctional HDL compared with strength-trained men irrespective of body weight status. J Appl Physiol 115(7):1043-9.

Millder WJ, et al. 1984. Effect of strength training on glucose tolerance and post-glucose insulin response. Med Sci Sports Exerc 16:539-43.

Layne JE, et al. 1999. The effect of progressive resistance training on bone density: a review. Med Sci Sports Exerc 31:25-30.

Moghadasi M, et al. 2012. The Effect of 12 Weeks of Resistance Training on hormones of Hone Formation in Young Sedentary women. Eur J Appl Physiol.

Koffler KH, et al. 1992. Strength training accelerates gastrointestinal transit in middle-aged and older men. Med Sci Sports Exerc.24:415-9.

Cuff DJ, et al. 2003. Effective exercise modality to reduce insulin resistance in women with type 2 diabetes. Diabetes Care 26 (11):2977-82.

Ross R, et al. 1994. Mobilization of visceral and sub- cutaneous adipose tissue in response to energy restriction and exercise. Am J Clin Nutr 60:695-703.

Ross R, et al. 1996. Influence of diet and exercise on skeletal muscle and visceral adipose tissue in men. J Appl Physiol 81:2445-55.

Rice B, et al. 1999. Effects of aerobic or resistance exercise and/or diet on glucose tolerance and plasma insulin levels in obese men. Diabetes Care 22:684-91.

Sundell J. 2011. Resistance training is an Effective Tool Against Metabolic and Frailty Syndromes. Advanced Preventative Medicine. 984683.

LaForgia J, et al. 2006. Effects of exercise intensity and duration on the excess post-exercise oxygen consumption. J Sports Sci 24:1247–1264.

Adams G, et al. 1993. Skeletal muscle myosin heavy chain composition and resistance training. Journal of Applied Physiology 74:911-15.

Evans WJ. 1999. Exercise training guidelines for the elderly. Med Sci Sports Exerc 31:12-7.

Ewart CK. 1989. Psychological effects of resistive weight training: implications for cardiac patients. Med Sci Sports Exerc 21:683-8.

Fragala MS. 2014. Resistance exercise may improve spatial awareness and visual reaction in older adults. J Strength Cond Res 28(8):2079-87.

Della Gatta PA, et al. 2014. Effect of exercise training on skeletal muscle cytokine expression in the elderly. Brain Behav Immun 39:80-86.

Carneiro NH, et al. 2015. Effects of difference resistance training frequencies on flexibility in older women. Clin Interv Aging 2015(10):531-538.

Booth FW, et al. 1997. Molecular events underlying skeletal muscle atrophy and the development of effective countermeasures. International Journal of Sports Medicine 18 (Suppl 4):S265-69.

Tang JE, et al. 2008. Resistance training alters the response of fed stated mixed muscle protein synthesis in young men. Am J Physiol Regul Integr Comp Physiol 294(1):R172-8.

Moore DR. 2014. Keeping older muscle "young" through dietary protein and physical activity. Adv Nutr 5(5):599S-607S.

Smutok MA, et al. 1993. Aerobic versus strength training for risk factor intervention in middle- aged men at high risk for coronary heart disease. Metabolism 42: 177-84.

Fitzgerald SJ, et al. 2004. Muscular fitness and all-cause mortality: prospective observations. J Physical Activity Health 1:7-18.

Black R. 1991. Muscle strength as an indicator of the habitual level of physical activity. Medicine and Science in Sports and Exercise 23:323-29.

Lowndes J, et al. 2009. Association of age with muscle size and strength before and after short-term resistance training in young adults. J Strength Cond Res 23(7):1915-20.

Mayhew DL, et al. 2009. Translational signaling responses preceding resistance training-mediated myofiber hypertrophy in young and old humans. J Appl Physiol 107:1655–1662.

Fiatarone MA, et al. 1990. High-intensity strength training in nonagenarians: Effect on skeletal muscle. JAMA 263-3029-34.

Churchward-Venne TA, et al. 2015. There are no nonresponders to resistance-type exercise training in older men and women. J Am Med Dir Assoc 16(5):400-11.

Dela F, et al. 2006. Resistance training, insulin sensitivity and muscle function in the elderly. Essays Biochem 42:75-88.

Brooks N, et al. 2007. Strength training improves muscle quality and insulin sensitivity in Hispanic older adults with type 2 diabetes. Int J Med Sci 4(1):19-27.

Eriksson J, et al. 1998. Aerobic endurance exercise or circuit-type resistance training for individuals with impaired glucose tolerance? Horm Metab Res 30(1):37-41.

Ishii T, 1998. et al. Resistance training improves insulin sensitivity in NIDDM subjects without altering maximal oxygen uptake. Diabetes Care 21(8):1353-5.

Ryan AS, et al. 2001. Insulin action after resistive training in insulin resistant older men and women. J Am Geriatr Soc 49(3):247-53.

Fenicchia LM, et al. 2004. Influence of resistance exercise training on glucose control in women with type 2 diabetes. Metabolism 53(3):284-9.

Ibanez J, et al. 2005. Twice-weekly progressive resistance training decreases abdominal fat and improves insulin sensitivity in older men with type 2 diabetes. Diabetes Care 28 (3):662-7.

Harridge SD, et al. 1999. Knee extensor strength, activation, and size in very elderly people following strength training. Muscle Nerve 22(7):831-9.

Kosek, D. J., et al., 2006. Efficacy of 3 days/wk resistance training on myofiber hypertrophy and myogenic mechanisms in young vs. older adults. J Appl Physiol 101:531-54.

Hagerman FC, et al. 2000. Effects of high-intensity resistance training on untrained older men I. Strength, cardiovascular, and metabolic responses. J Geront Series A, Biol Sci Med Sci 55(7):B336–46.

Harris C, et al. 2004. The effect of resistance-training intensity on strength-gain response in the older adult. J Strength Cond Res 18(4):833–8.

Narici MV, et al. 2004. Muscular adaptations to resistance exercise in the elderly. Journal of Musculoskeletal & Neuronal Interactions 4(2):161–4.

Roth, S. M., et al., 2003. Myostatin gene expression is reduced in humans with heavy-resistance strength training: a brief communication. Exp Biol Med 228:706-9.

Miszko TA, et al. 2003. Effect of strength and power training on physical function in community-dwelling older adults. J Geront Series A, Biol Sci Med Sci 58(2):171–5.

Porter MM. 2006. Power training for older adults. Appl Physiol Nutr Metab (2):87–94.

Adams KJ, et al., 1992. The effect of six weeks of squat, plyometric and squat-plyometric training on power production. J Appl Sports Sci Res 6:36-41.

Sihvonen S, et al. 2004. Fall incidence in frail older women after individualized visual feedback-based balance training. Gerontology 50: 411–416.

Principle #3

Beckham S, et al. 2010. Functional training: Fad or here to stay? ACSM's Health & Fitness Journal 14(6):24-30.

Carson RG. 2006. Changes in muscle coordination with training. J Appl Physiol 101(5):1506-13.

Schoenfeld B. 2010. Is functional training really functional? ACSM Certified News. 20(3), 5-6, 2010.

Kraemer WJ, et al. 2002. American College of Sports Medicine position stand. Progression models in resistance training for healthy adults. Med Sci Sports Exerc 34:364–380.

Kraemer WJ, et al. 2004. Fundamentals of resistance training: progression and exercise prescription. Med Sci Sports Exerc 36:674–688.

Hansen, S, et al. 2001. The effect of short-term strength training on human skeletal muscle: The importance of physiologically elevated hormone levels. Scan J Med Sci Sport 11:347–354.

Kraemer WJ, et al. 1992. Acute hormonal responses in elite junior weightlifters. Int J Sport Med 13:103–109.

Chilibeck PD, et al. 1998. A comparison of strength and muscle mass increases during resistance training in young women. Eur J Appl Physiol 77:170-5.

McCaw ST, et al. 1994. A comparison of muscle activity between a free weight and machine bench press. J Strength Cond Res 8:259-64.

Shaner AA, et al. 2014. The acute hormonal response to free weight and machine weight resistance exercise. J Strength Cond Res 28:1032-1040.

Black A, et al. 2012. Hormonal Response to Free Eight and Machine Weight Resistance Exercise. Eighth International Conference on Strength Training. Norway: Oslo.

Nisell R, et al. 1986. Joint load during the parallel squat in powerlifting and force analysis of in vivo bilateral quadriceps tendon rupture. Scan J Sport Sci 8: 63–70.

Stoppani, J. Encyclopedia of Muscle and Strength. Champaign, IL: Human Kinetics Publishers, 2006. Pg 151.

Stone M, et al. 1979. A short-term comparison of two different methods of resistance training on leg strength and power. Athletic Training 14:158-60.

Croisier JL, et al. 2008. Strength imbalances and prevention of hamstring injury in professional soccer players: a prospective study. Am J Sports Med,36(8):1469-75.

Willoughby GS, et al. 1990. A comparison of isotonic free weights and omnikinetic exercise machines on strength. J Human Mov Stud 19:93-100.

Clark D, et al. 2012. Muscle Activation in the Loaded Free Barbell Squat: A Brief Review. J Strength Cond Res 26(4):1169-1178.

Comfort P, et al. 2011. An Electromyographical Comparison of Trunk Muscle activity During Isometric Trunk and Dynamic Strengthening Exercises. J Strength Cond Res 2591:149-154.

Ronei P, et al. 2012. Effect of Range of Motion on Muscle Strength and Thickness. J Strength Cond Res 26(8):2140-2145.

Goldspink G. 2002. Gene expression in skeletal muscle. Biochem Soc Trans 30:285–290.

Hornberger TA, et al. 2006. Mechanical stimuli and nutrients regulate rapamycin-sensitive signaling through distinct mechanisms in skeletal muscle. J Cell Biochem 97:1207–1216.

Vandenburgh HH. 1987. Motion into mass: How does tension stimulate muscle growth? Med Sci Sport Exerc 19(5 Suppl.):S142–S149.

O'Sullivan K, et al. 2012. The Effects of Eccentric Graining on Lower Limb Flexibility: A Review. Brit J Sports Med.

Principle #4

Colado J, et al. 2011. The Progression of Paraspinal Muscle Recruitment Intensity in Localized and Global Strength Training Exercise is not Based on Instability Alone. Arch Phys Med Rehab 92:1875-1883.

Escamilla RF, et al. 2002. An electromyographic analysis of sumo and conventional style deadlifts. Med Sci Sports Exerc 34(4):682-8.

Contreras B. "Hip and Glute Thrust Science." Bret Contreras: The Glute Guy. 6 Apr. 2013. <http://bretcontreras.com/hip-thrust-and-glute-science/>.

Worrell TW, et al. 2001. Influence of joint position on electromyographic and torque generation during maximal voluntary isometric contractions of the hamstrings and gluteus maximus muscles. J Orthop Sports Phys Ther 31(12):730-40.

Contreras BM, et al. 2013. Are all hip extension exercises created equal? Strength Cond J 35(2):17-22.

Beardsley CM, et al. 2014. The increasing role of the hip extensor musculature with heavier compound lower-body movements and more explosive sport actions. Strength Cond J 36(2):49-55.

Bryanton MA, et al. 2012. Effect of squat depth and barbell load on relative muscular effort in squatting. J Strength Cond Res 26(10):2820-8.

Riemann BL, et al. 2012. Biomechanical analysis of the Anterior lunge during 4 external-load Conditions. J Athletic Train 47:372–378.

Swinton PA, et al. 2011. A biomechanical analysis of straight and hexagonal barbell deadlifts using submaximal loads. J Strength Cond Res 25:2000–2009.

Schache AG, et al. 2011. Effect of running speed on lower limb joint kinetics. Med Sci Sports Exerc 43:1260.

Lees A, et al. 2004. The maximal and submaximal vertical jump: Implications for strength and conditioning. J Strength Cond Res 18:787–791.

Buśko K, et al. 2011. Muscle strength and power of elite female and male swimmers. Baltic J Health Phys Activity 3:13–18.

McLaughlin TM, et al. 1978. Kinetics of the parallel squat. Res Q 49:175–189, 1978.

Miletello WM, et al. 2009. A biomechanical analysis of the squat between competitive collegiate, competitive high school, and novice powerlifters. J Strength Cond Res 23:1611–1617.

Myer GD, et al. 2011. Real-time assessment and neuromuscular training feedback techniques to prevent ACL injury in female athletes. Strength Cond J 33:21–35.

Myer GD, et al. 2014. The Back Squat: A proposed assessment of functional deficits and technical factors that limit performance Strength Cond J 36(6):4-27.

Brocki KC, et al. 2004. Executive functions in children aged 6 to 13: A dimensional and developmental study. Dev Neuropsychol 26:571–593.

Escamilla RF. 2001. Knee biomechanics of the dynamic squat exercise. Med Sci Sports Exerc 33: 127–141.

Yavus HU, et al. 2014. Kinematic and EMG activities during front and back squat variations in maximum loads. J Sport Sci 33(10):1058-1066.

Gullet JC, et al. 2009. A biomechanical comparison of back and front squats in healthy trained indviduals. J Strength Cond Res 23(1):284-92.

Bell R. "The Best Kept Secret: Why People Have to Squat Differently." The Movement Fix. 9 Jan 2014. <http://themovementfix.com/the-best-kept-secret-why-people-have-to-squat-differently/>.

Youdas, J., et al. 2010. Surface Electromyographic Activation Patterns and Elbow Joint Motion During a Pull-Up, Chin-Up or Perfect-Pull-up Rotational Exercise. J Strength Cond Res 24(12):3404-3414.

DiNubile N. 1991. Strength training. Clin Sport Med 10:33-63.

Ebben W, et al. 2011. Kinetic Analysis of Several Variations of Push-Ups. J Strength Cond Res 25(10):2891-2894.

McCurdy KW, et al. 2005. The effects of short-term unilateral and bilateral lower-body resistance training on measures of strength and power. J Strength Cond Res 19:9-15.

Shirey M, et al. 2012. The Influence of Core Musculature Engagement on Hip and Knee Kinematics in Women during a Single-Leg Squat. Inter J Sport Phys Therap 7(1):1-12.

Jones M, et al. 2012. Effects of Unilateral and Bilateral Lower-Body Heavy Resistance Exercise on Muscle Activity and Testosterone Response. J Strength Cond Res.

Spreuwenberg LP, et al. 2006. Influence of exercise order in a resistance-training exercise session. J Strength Cond Res 20:141-4.

ACSM. 2009. American College of Sports Medicine position stand. Progression models in resistance training for healthy adults. Med Sci Sports Exerc 41(3):687-708.

McGill S. 2010. Core Training: Evidence Translating to Better Performance and Injury Prevention. Strength Cond J 32(3), 33-46.

Richardson C, et al. 1999. Therapeutic exercise for spinal segmental stabilization in low back pain: Scientifi c basis and clinical approach. Edinburgh, NY: Churchill Livingstone.

Fig G. 2005. Sport-specifi c conditioning: strength training for swimmers—Training the core. Strength Cond J 27(2):40–41.

Gottschall JS, et al. 2013. Integration core exercises elicit greater muscle activation than isolation exercises. J Strength Cond Res 27(3):590-6.

Jackson A, et al. 1985. Strength development: using functional isometrics in an isotonic strength training program. Res Q Exerc Sport 56:234-7.

McGill SM. 2001. Low back stability: from formal description to issues for performance and rehabilitation. Exerc Sports Sci Rev 29:26-31.

Contreras B, et al. 2011. To crunch or not to crunch: An evidence-based examination of spinal flexion exercises, their potential risks, and their applicability to program design. Strength Cond J 33(4):8–18.

Zheng N, et al. 2008. Kinematic analysis of swing in pro and amateur golfers. Int J Sports Med 29(6):487–493.

Principle #5

Gentilcore, T. "5 Major Benefits of Total-Body Workouts - Life by DailyBurn." Life by DailyBurn 5 Major Benefits of TotalBody Workouts Comments. 04 Nov. 2014. <http://dailyburn.com/life/fitness/benefits-total-body-workout/>.

Cumming DC, et al. 1986. Reproductive hormone increases in response to acute exercise in men. Med Sci Sports Exerc 18(4):369-73.

Kraemer WJ, et al. 2005. Hormonal Responses and Adaptations to Resistance Exercise & Training. Sports Med 35:339-361.

Villanueva M, et al. 2012. Acute Hormonal Responses to Various Resistance Training Schemes. J Strength Cond Res.

Alcaraz P, et al. 2011. Similarity in Adaptations to high-Resistance Circuit Vs. Traditional Strength Training in Resistance-Trained Men. J Strength Cond Res 25(9):2519-2525.

Parinatti P, et al. 2011.The Effect of Between-Set Rest Intervals on the Oxygen Uptake During and After Resistance Exercise Sessions Performed with Large- and Small-Muscle Mass. J Strength Cond Res 25(11):3181-3187.

Vandenburgh HH, et al. 1987. Motion into mass: How does tension stimulate muscle growth? Med Sci Sport Exerc 19(5 Suppl):S142–S149.

Goldberg, AL, et al. 1975. Mechanism of work-induced hypertrophy of skeletal muscle. Med Sci Sport Exerc 7:185–198.

Evans, WJ. 2002. Effects of exercise on senescent muscle. Clin Orthopaed Rel Res 403(Suppl.): S211–S220.

Toigo M, et al. 2006. New fundamental resistance exercise determinants of molecular and cellular muscle adaptations. Eur J Appl Physiol 97:643–663.

Vierck J, et al. 2000. Satellite cell regulation following myotrauma caused by resistance exercise. Cell Biol Int 24:263–272.

Crewther B, et al. 2006. Possible stimuli for strength and power adaptation: Acute hormonal responses. Sport Med 36:215–238.

Deschenes MR, et al. 1991. Exercise induced hormonal changes and their effects upon skeletal muscle muscle tissue. Sport Med 12:80–89.

McCall GE, et al. 1996. Muscle fiber hypertrophy, hyperplasia, and capillary density in college men after resistance training. J Appl Physiol 81:2004-12.

Rooney KJ, et al. 1994. Fatigue contributes to the strength training stimulus. Med Sci Sport Exerc 26:1160–1164.

Schott, J, et al. 1995. The role of metabolites in strength training. II. Short versus long isometric contractions. Eur J Appl Physiol 71:337–341.

Smith RC, et al. 1995. The role of metabolites in strength training. I. A comparison of eccentric and concentric contractions. Eur J Appl Physiol Occup Physiol 71:332–336.

Schoenfeld B. 2010. The mechanisms of muscle hypertrophy and their application to resistance training. J Strength Cond Res 24(10):2857-2872.

Buchtal F, et al. 1970. Contraction times and fiber type in intact human muscle. Acta Physiol Scand 79:435-40.

Robbins DW, et al. Effects of agonist-antagonist complex resistance training on upper body strength and power development. J Sports Sci 27(14):1617-25.

Baker D, et al. Acute effect on power output of alternating an agonist and antagonist muscle exercise during complex training. J Strength Cond Res 19(1):202-5.

Macintosh, A. "From Athletes to Couch Potatoes: Humans through 6,000 Years of Farming." University of Cambridge. 8 Apr. 2014.

Ronnestad B, et al. 2011. Physiological Elevation of Endogenous Hormones Results in superior Strength training Adaptation. Eur J Appl Physiol 111:2249-2259.

Migiano M, et al. 2010. Endocrine Response Patterns to Acute Unilateral and Bilateral Resistance Exercise in Men. J Strength Cond Res 24(8):128-134.

Calder AW, et al. 1994. Comparison of whole and split weight training routines in young women. Can J Appl Physiol 19(2):185-99.

Benton MJ, et al. 2011. Short-term effects of resistance training frequency on body composition and strength in middle-aged women. J Strength Cond Res 25(11):3142-9.

Simao R, et al. 2007. Influence of exercise order on the number of repetitions performed and perceived exertion during resistance exercise in women. J Strength Cond Res 21:23-8.

Soncin et al. 2014. Influence of exercise order on electromyographic activity during upper body resistance training. J Human Kin.

Principle #6

Rhea MR, et al. 2003. A meta-analysis to determine the dose response for strength development. Med Sci Sports Exerc 35:456-64.

Coburn JW, et al. 2006. Neuromuscular responses to three days of velocity-specific isokinetic training. J Strength Cond Res 20:892-8.

Weiss LW, et al. 1999. Differential functional adaptations to short-term low-, moderate-, and high-repetition weight training. J Strength Cond Res 13(3).

Chestnut JL, et al. 1999. The effects of 4 and 10 repetition maximum weight-training protocols on neuromuscular adaptations in untrained men. J Strength Cond Res 13(4).

O'Shea P. 2013. Effects of selected weight training programs on the development of strength and muscle hypertrophy. Exerc Sport 37(1):95-102.

Holm L, et al. 2008. Changes in muscle size and MHC composition in response to resistance exercise with heavy and light loading intensity. J Appl Physiol 105:1454–1461.

Campos GE, et al. 2002. Muscular adaptations in response to three different resistance-training regimens: specificity of repetition maximum training zones. Eur J Appl Physiol 88:50-60.

Staron RS, et al. 1994. Skeletal muscle adaptations during early phase of heavy-resistance training in men and women. J Appl Physiol 76:1247-55.

ACSM. 2009. American College of Sports Medicine position stand. Progression models in resistance training for healthy adults. Med Sci Sports Exerc 41(3):687-708.

Berger RA. 1962. Optimum repetitions for the development of strength. Res Q 33:334-8.

O'Shea P. 1966. Effects of selected weight training programs on the development of strength and muscle hypertrophy. Res Q 37:95-102.

Willardson JM. 2007. The application of training to failure in periodized multiple-set resistance exercise programs. J Strength Cond Res 21:628–631.

Rooney KJ, et al. 1994. Fatigue contributes to the strength training stimulus. Med Sci Sport Exerc 26: 1160–1164.

Linnamo V, et al. 2005. Acute hormonal responses to submaximal and maximal high intensity resistance and explosive exercise in men and women. J Strength Cond Res 19, 566–571.

Sampson JA, et al. 2015. Is repetition failure critical for the development of muscle hypertrophy and strength? Med Sci Sport.

Fry AC, et al. 1997. Resistance exercise overtraining and overreaching: Neuroendocrine responses. Sport Med 23:106–129.

Izquierdo M. et al. 2006. Differential effects of strength training leading to failure versus not to failure on hormonal responses, strength and muscle power increases. J Appl Physiol 100:1647–1656.

Farthing JP, et al. 2003. The effects of eccentric and concentric training at different velocities on muscle hypertrophy. Eur J Appl Physiol 89:578–586.

Higbie EJ, et al. 1996. Effects of concentric and eccentric training on muscle strength, crosssectional area, and neural activation. J Appl Physiol 81:2173–2181.

Hortobagyi T, et al. 1996. Greater initial adaptations to submaximal muscle lengthening than maximal shortening. J Appl Physiol 81:1677–1682.

Seger JY, et al. 1998. Specific effects of eccentric and concentric training on muscle strength and morphology in humans. Eur J Appl Physiol Occup Physiol 79(1):49-57.

Hortobagyi T, et al. 1996. Adaptive responses to muscle lengthening and shortening in humans. J Appl Physiol 80(3):765-72.

Vikne H, et al. 2006. Muscular performance after concentric and eccentric exercise in trained men. Med Sci Sports Exerc 38(10):1770-81.

Hortobagyi T, et al. 2000. Changes in muscle strength, muscle fiber size and myofibrillar gene expression after immobilization. J Physiol 524(pt 1):293-304.

Bonde-Peterson F, et al. 1972. Muscle metabolism during exercise with concentric and eccentric contractions. J Appl Physiology 33:792-5.

Komi PV, et al. EMG activity of leg extensor muscles with special reference to mechanical efficiency in concentric and eccentric exercise. Int J Sports Med 8(Suppl):22-9.

Roig M, et al. 2009. The effects of eccentric versus concentric resistance training on muscle strength and mass in healthy adults: a systematic review with meta-analysis. Br J Sports Med 43(8):556-68.

Moore DR, et al. 2005. Myofibrillar and collagen protein synthesis in human skeletal muscle in young men after maximal shortening and lengthening contractions. Am J Physiol Endocrinol Metab 288:E1153–E1159.

Shepstone TN, et al. 2005. Short-term high- vs. low-velocity isokinetic lengthening training results in greater hypertrophy of the elbow flexors in young men. J Appl Physiol 98:1768–1776.

Bentley J, et al. 2010. Effect of Different Lifting Cadences on Ground Reaction Forces During the Squat Exercise. J Strength Cond Res 24(5):1414-1420.

McHugh MP, et al. 2000. Electromyographic analysis of exercise resulting in symptoms of muscle damage. J Sport Sci 18:163–172.

Ebbeling CB, et al. 1989. Exercise-induced muscle damage and adaptation. Sports Med
7:207-34.

Neto et al. 2012. Long-Term Adaptations Differ for Shortening and Lengthening Contractions. Eur J Appl Physiol 112:3709-3720.

Hather BM, et al. 1991. Influence of eccentric actions on skeletal muscle adaptations to resistance training. Acta Physiol Scand 143:177-85.

Pareja-Blanco F, et al. 2014. Effect of movement velocity during resistance training on neuromuscular performance. Int J Sports Med 35(11):916-24.

Keeler LK, et al. 2001. Early-phase adaptations of traditional-speed vs. SuperSlow resistance training on strength and aerobic capacity in sedentary individuals. J Strength Cond Res 15:309–314.

Neils CM, et al. 2005. Influence of contraction velocity in untrained individuals over the initial early phase of resistance training. J Strength Cond Res 19:883–887.

Nogueira W, et al. 2009. Effects of power training on muscle thickness of older men. Int J Sport Med 30:200–204.

Behm DG, et al. 1993. Intended rather than actual movement velocity determines the velocity-specific training response. J Appl Physiol 74:359-68.

Faulker J. et al. 1986. Power output of fast and slow fibers from human skeletal muscles. In Human Muscle Power, ed. 81-90. Champaign, IL: Human Kinetics

Lexell J, et al. 1992. What is the effect of aging on type 2 muscle fibers? J Neurol Sci 107:250-1.

Hakkinen K., et al. 2001. Changes in electromyographic activity, muscle fibre and force production characteristics during heavy resistance/power strength training in middle-aged and older men and women. Acta Physiol Scand 171:51-62.

Tsourlou T, et al. 2006. The effects of a twenty-four-week aquatic training program on muscular strength performance in healthy elderly women. J Strength Cond Res 20:811-8.

Lexell J. 1995. Human aging, muscle mass, and fiber type composition. J Gerontol A Biol Sci Med Sci 50A:11–16.

Trappe S, et al. 2003. Single muscle fiber contractile properties in young and old men and women. J Physiol 552:47–58.

Whipple RH, et al. 1987. The relationship of knee and ankle weakness to falls in nursing home residents: an isokinetic study. J Am Geriatr Soc 35:13–20.

Pijnappels M, et al. 2008. Identification of elderly fallers by muscle strength measures. Eur J Appl Physiol 102:585-92.

Claflin DR, et al. 2011. Effects of high- and low-velocity resistance training on the contractile properties of skeletal muscle fibers from young and older humans. J Appl Physiol 111(4):1021-1030.

Bottaro M, et al. 2007. Effect of high versus low-velocity resistance training on muscular fitness and functional performance in older men. Eur J Appl Physiol 99:257–264.

Fielding RA, et al. 2002. High-velocity resistance training increases skeletal muscle peak power in older women. J Am Geriatr Soc 50:655–662.

Marsh AP, et al. 2009. Lower extremity muscle function after strength or power training in older adults. J Aging Phys Act 17:416–443.

Sayers SP. 2008. High velocity power training in older adults. Curr Aging Sci 1:62–67.

De Vos NJ, et al. 2005. Optimal load for increasing muscle power during explosive resistance training in older adults. J Gerontol 60A:638-47.

Kawamori N, et al. 2004. The optimal training load for the development of muscular power. J Strength Cond Res 18:675-84.

Tanimoto M, et al. 2006. Effects of low-intensity resistance exercise with slow movement and tonic force generation on muscular function in young men. J Appl Physiol 100(4):1150-1157.

Young WB, et al. 1993. The effect of voluntary effort to influence speed of contraction on strength, muscular power, and hypertrophy development. J Strength Cond Res 7(3).

Hunter GR, et al. 2003. Comparison of metabolic and heart rate responses to super slow vs. traditional resistance training. J Strength Cond Res 17:76-81.

Lachance PF, et al. 1994. Influence of cadence on muscular performance during push-up and pull-up exercises. J Strength Cond Res 8:76-9.

Ratamess NA, et al. 2007. The effect of rest interval length on metabolic responses to the bench press exercise. Eur J Appl Physiol 100:1-17.

Kraemer WJ, et al. 2005. Hormonal responses and adaptations to resistance exercise and training. Sports Med 35:339-61.

Goto, K, et al. 2004. Muscular adaptations to combinations of high- and low-intensity resistance exercises. J Strength Cond Res 18:730–737.

Miranda H, et al. 2007. Effect of two different rest period lengths on the number of repetitions performed during resistance training. J Strength Cond Res 21:1032–1036.

Richmond SR, et al. 2004. The effects of varied rest periods between sets to failure using the bench press in recreationally trained men. J Strength Cond Res 18:846-9.

Willardson JM, et al. 2005. A comparison of 3 different rest intervals on the exercise volume completed during a workout. J Strength Cond Res 19:23-6.

Willardson JM, et al. 2006. The effect of rest interval length on the sustainability of squat and bench press repetitions. J Strength Cond Res 20:400-3.

Celes R, et al. 2010. Gender muscule recovery during isokinetic exercise. Int J Sports Med 31(12):866-9.

Bottaro M, et al. 2010. Effects of age and rest interval on strength recovery. Int J Sports Med 31(1):22-5.

Theou O, et al. Effect of rest interval on strength recovery in young and old women. J Strength Cond Res 22(6):1876-81.

Parcell AC, et al. 2002. Minimum rest period for strength recovery during a common isokinetic testing protocol. Med Sci Sports Exerc 34(6):1018-22.

Pincivero D, et al. 1997. Effects of rest interval on isokinetic strength and functional performance after short term high intensity training. Br J Sports Med 31:229-34.

Schoenfeld BJ. 2013. Potential mechanisms for a role of metabolic stress in hypertrophic adaptations in resistance training. Sports Med 43(3):179-94.

de Salles BF, et al. 2009. Rest interval between sets in strength training. Sport Med 39:765–777.

Kraemer WJ, et al. 1990. Hormonal and growth factor responses to heavy resistance exercise protocols. J Appl Physiol 69:1442–1450.

Kraemer WJ, et al. 1991. Endogenous anabolic hormonal and growth factor responses to heavy resistance exercise in males and females. Int J Sport Med 12:228–235.

Hoffman JR, et al. 2003. Effect of muscle oxygenation during resistance exercise on anabolic hormone response. Med Sci Sport Exerc 35:1929–1934.

Kraemer WJ, et al. 1993. Effects of different heavy-resistance exercise protocols on plasma beta-endorphin concentrations. J Appl Physiol (1985) 74(1):450-9.

Rhea MR, et al. 2002. Single versus multiple sets for strength: a meta-analysis to address the controversary. Res Q Exerc Sport 75:413-22.

Galvao D, et al. 2004. Single vs. multiple-set resistance training: Recent developments in the controversary. J Strength Cond Res 18:660-67.

Radaelli R, et al. 2015. Dose-response of 1, 3, and 5 sets of resistance exercise on strength, local muscular endurance, and hypertrophy. J Strength Cond Res 29(5):1349-1358.

Wolfe BL, et al. 2004. Quantitative analysis of single- vs. multiple-set programs in resistance training. J Strength Cond Res 18:35–47.

Burd NA, et al. 2010. Resistance exercise volume affects myofibrillar protein synthesis and anabolic signalling molecule phosphorylation in young men. J Physiol 588:3119–3130.

Ronnestad BR, et al. 2007. Dissimilar effects of one-and three-set training on strength and muscle mass gains in upper and lower body in untrained subjects. J Strength Cond Res 21:157-63.

Kraemer WJ, et al. 2000. Influence of resistance training volume and periodization on physiological and performance adaptations in college women tennis players. Am J Sports 28:626-33.

Marx JO, et al. 2001. The effects of single-set vs. periodized multiple-set resistance training on muscular performance and hormonal concentrations in women. Med Sci Sports Exerc 33:635-43.

Oates BR, et al. 2010. Low-volume resistance exercise attenuates the decline in strength and muscle mass associated with immobilization. Muscle Nerve 42:539–546.

Krieger JW. 2010. Single vs. multiple sets of resistance exercise for muscle hypertrophy: a meta-analysis. J Strength Cond Res 24(4):1150-9.

Craig B, et al. 1994. Growth hormone release following single versus multiple sets of back squats: Total work versus power. J Strength Cond Res 8:270–275.

Mulligan SE, et al. 1996. Influence of resistance exercise volume on serum growth hormone and cortisol concentrations in women. J Strength Cond Res 10:256–262.

Smilios I, et al. 2003. Hormonal responses after various resistance exercise protocols. Med Sci Sport Exerc 35:644–654.

Schwab R, et al. 1993. Acute effects of different intensities of weight lifting on serum testosterone. Med Sci Sport Exerc 25:1381–1385.

Kemmler WK, et al. 2004. Effects of single- vs. multiple-set resistance training on maximum strength and body composition in trained postmenopausal women. J Strength Cond Res 18:689-94.

Ostrowski KJ, et al. 1997. The effect of weight training volume on hormonal output and muscular size and function. J Strenght Cond Res 11:148-54.

Capen EK. 1956. Study of four programs of heavy resistance exercises for development of muscular strength. Res Q 27:132-42.

Berger RA. 1962. Effect of varied weight training programs on strength. Res Q 168-81.

Ploutz LL, et al. 1994. Effect of resistance training on muscle use during exercise. J Apply Physiol 76:1675-81.

Rhea MR, et al. 2004. A meta-analysis of periodized versus nonperiodized strength and power training programs. Res Quart Exerc Sport 75(4):413-22.

Fleck SJ and Kraemer WJ. 1997. Designing Resistance Training Programs. 2nd ed. Champaign (IL): Human Kinetics Books.

Kraemer WJ, et al. Fundamentals of resistance training: progression and exercise prescription. Med Sci Sports Exerc 36:674-8.

Sale DG. 1992. Neural adaptations to strength training. In: Komi, P. V. Strength and Power in Sport. Oxford: Blackwell Scientific, pg. 249-65.

Fleck SJ, et al. 1988. Cardiovascular adaptations to resistance training. Med Sci Sports Exerc 20:S146-51.

Dolezal BA, et al. 1998. Concurrent resistance and endurance training influence basal metabolic rate in nondieting individuals. J Appl Physiol. 85:695-700.

Hakkinen K, et al. 1998. Changes in agonist-antagonist EMG, muscle CSA, and force during strength training in middle-aged and older people. J Appl Physiol 84:1341-9.

Fleck SJ. 1999. Periodized strength training: a critical review. J Strength Cond Res 13:82-9.

Hakkinen K, et al. 1987. Relationships between training volume, physical performance capacity, and serum hormone concentrations during prolonged training in elite weight lifters. Int J Sports Med 8(suppl):61-5.

Principle #7

ACSM. 2009. American College of Sports Medicine position stand. Progression models in resistance training for healthy adults. Med Sci Sports Exerc 41(3):687-708.

Feigenbaum MS, et al. 1999. Prescription of resistance training for health and disease. Med Sci Sports Exerc 31:38-45.

Focht BC. 2007. Perceived exertion and training load during self-selected and imposed-intensity resistance exercise in untrained women. J Strength Cond Res 21:183-7.

Glass S, et al. 2004. Self-selected resistance training intensity in novice weightlifters. J Strength Cond Res 18:324-7.

Campos GE, et al. 2002. Muscular adaptations in response to three different resistancetraining regimens: Specificity of repetition maximum training zones. Eur J Appl Physiol 88:50–60.

Kerksick CM, et al. 2009. Early-phase adaptations to a split-body, linear periodization resistance training program in college-aged and middle-aged men. J Strength Cond Res 23:962–971.

Robergs RA, et al. 2003. Biochemistry of exercise induced metabolic acidosis. Am J Physiol. Reg Int Comp Physiol 287:R502–R516.

Esse´n-Gustavsson B, et al. 1990. Glycogen and triglyceride utilization in relation to muscle metabolic characteristics in men performing heavy-resistance exercise. Eur J Appl Physiol Occupl Physiol 61:5–10.

Tesch PA, et al. 1986. Muscle metabolism during intense, heavy-resistance exercise. Eur J Appl Physiol Occup Physiol 55:362–366.

Willardson JM. 2007. The application of training to failure in periodized multiple-set resistance exercise programs. J Strength Cond Res 21:628–631.

Hakkinen K, et al. 1993. Acute hormonal responses to two different fatiguing heavy-resistance protocols in male athletes. J Appl Physiol 74: 882–887.

Kraemer WJ, et al. 1993. Changes in hormonal concentrations after different heavy resistance exercise protocols in women. J Appl Physiol 75:594–604.

Kraemer WJ, et al. 1991. Endogenous anabolic hormonal and growth factor responses to heavy resistance exercise in males and females. Int J Sport Med 12:228–235.

Kraemer WJ, et al. 1990. Hormonal and growth factor responses to heavy resistance exercise protocols. J Appl Physiol 69:1442–1450.

McCaulley GO, et al. 2009. Acute hormonal and neuromuscular responses to hypertrophy, strength and power type resistance exercise. Eur J Appl Physiol 105:695–704.

Suga T, et al. 2009. Intramuscular metabolism during low-intensity resistance exercise with blood flow restriction. J Appl Physiol 106:1119–1124.

Gordon SE, et al. 1994. Effect of acid–base balance on the growth hormone response to acute high-intensity cycle exercise. J Appl Physiol 76:821–829.

Goto K, et al. 2005. The impact of metabolic stress on hormonal responses and muscular adaptations. Med Sci Sport Exerc 37:955–963.

Takarada Y, et al. 2000. Rapid increase in plasma growth hormone after lowintensity resistance exercise with vascular occlusion. J Appl Physiol 88:61–65.

Kraemer WJ, et al. 1987. Physiological responses to heavy-resistance exercise with very short rest periods. Int J Sports Med 8:247-52.

Shinohara M, et al. 1998. Efficacy of tourniquet ischemia for strength training with low resistance. Eur J Appl Physiol 77:189–191.

Weiss LW, et al. 1999. Differential functional adaptations to short-term low- moderate-, and high-repetition weight training. J Strength Cond Res 13:236-41.

Burd NA, et al. 2010. Low-load high volume resistance exercise stimulates muscle protein synthesis more than high-load low volume resistance exercise in young men. PLoS One 5:e12033.

Mitchell CJ, et al. 2012. Resistance exercise load does not determine training-mediated hypertrophic gains in young men. J Appl Physiol 113(1):71-77.

Barcelos LC, et al. 2015. Low-load resistance training promotes muscular adaptation regardless of vascular occlusion, load, or volume. Eur J Appl Physiol 115(7):1559-1568.

Schoenfeld BJ. 2013. Is there a minimum intensity threshold for resistance training-induced hypertrophic adaptations? Sports Med 43(12):1279-1288.

Hakkinen K, et al. 1985. Changes in isometric force-and relaxation-time, electromyographic and muscle fibre characteristics of human skeletal muscle during strength training and detraining. Acta Physiol Scand 125:587-600.

Carneiro NH, et al. 2015. Effects of different resistance training frequencies on flexibility in older women. 2015(10):531-538.

Bloomquist K, et al. 2013. Effect of range of motion in heavy load squatting on muscle and tendon adaptations. Eur J Appl Physiol 113(8):2133-42.

McDonagh MJN, et al. 1984. Adaptive response of mammalian skeletal muscle to exercise with high loads. Eur J Appl Physiol 52:139–155.

Szivak T., Hooper, D., et al. Adrenal Cortical Responses to High Intensity, Short Rest, Resistance Exercise in Men and Women. Journal of Strength and Conditioning Research. 2012.

Hakkinen K, et al. 1991. Serum hormones in male strength athletes during intensive short term strength training. Eur J Appl Physiol 63:191–199.

Raastad, T, et al. 2001. Changes in human skeletal muscle contractility and hormone status during 2 weeks of heavy strength training. Eur J Appl Physiol 84:54–63.

Fry AC, et al. 1997. Resistance exercise overtraining and overreaching: Neuroendocrine responses. Sport Med 23:106–129.

Hakkinen, KA, et al. 1987. Relationships between training volume, physical performance capacity, and serum hormone concentrations during prolonged training in elite weight lifters. Int J Sport Med 8(Suppl.):61–65.

Micheli L. 1988. Injuries and prolonged exercise. In Prolonged Exercise, ed. D. Lamb and R. Murray, 393-407. Indianopolis: Benchmark Press.

Rhea MR, et al. 2004. A meta-analysis of periodized versus nonperiodized strength and power training programs. Res Q Exerc Sport. 75:413-22.

Principle #8

Hood D, et al. 1990. Amino acid metabolism during exercise and following endurance training. Sports Med 9:23-25.

Lemon P, et al. 1980. Effect of initial glycogen levels on protein metabolism during exercise. J Appl Physiol 71:404-9.

Lemon P, et al. 1980. Effects of exercise on protein and amino acid metabolism. Med Sci Sports Exerc 13:141-49.

Pasiakos SM, et al. 2014. Effects of protein supplements on muscle damage, soreness and recovery of muscle function and physical performance: a systematic review. Sports Med 44(5):655-70.

Rahbek SK, et al. 2015. No differential effects of divergent isocaloric supplements on signalling for muscle protein turnover during recovery from muscle-damaging eccentric exercise. Amino Acids 47(4):767-778.

Chesley A, et al. 1992. Changes in human muscle protein synthesis after resistance exercise. J Appl Physiol 73:1383–1388.

Biolo G, et al. 1995. Increased rates of muscle protein turnover and amino acid transport after resistance exercise in humans. Am J Physiol Endocrinol Metab 268:E514–E520.

Phillips SM, et al. 1997. Mixed muscle protein synthesis and breakdown after resistance exercise in humans. Am J Physiol Endocrinol Metab 273:E99–E107.

Dreyer HC, et al. 2006. Exercise increases AMPK activity and reduces 4E-BP1 phosphorylation and protein synthesis in human skeletal muscle. J Physiol 576:613–624.

Wilkinson SB, et al. 2008. Differential effects of resistance and endurance exercise in the fed state on signalling molecule phosphorylation and protein synthesis in human muscle. J Physiol 586:3701–3717.

Devries MC, et al. 2015. Supplemental protein in support of muscle mass and health: advantage whey. J Food Sci 80(S1):A8-A15.

Rennie MJ, et al. 2004. Control of the size of the human muscle mass. Annu Rev Physiol 66:799–828.

Cermak NM, et al. 2012. Protein supplementation augments the adaptive response of skeletal muscle to resistance-type exercise training: a meta-analysis. Am J Clin Nutr 96:1454–1464.

West DW, et al. 2010. Elevations in ostensibly anabolic hormones with resistance exercise enhance neither training-induced muscle hypertrophy nor strength of the elbow flexors. J Appl Physiol 108:60–67.

Hartman JW, et al. 2007. Consumption of fat-free fluid milk after resistance exercise promotes greater lean mass accretion than does consumption of soy or carbohydrate in young, novice, male weightlifters. Am J Clin Nutr 86:373–381.

West DW, et al. 2009. Resistance exercise-induced increases in putative anabolic hormones do not enhance muscle protein synthesis or intracellular signalling in young men. J Physiol 587:5239–5247.

MacDougall JD, et al. 1995. The time course for elevated muscle protein synthesis following heavy resistance exercise. Can J Appl Physiol 20:480-6.

Burd NA, et al. 2009. Exercise training and protein metabolism: influences of contraction, protein intake, and sex-based differences. J Appl Physiol 106(5):1692-1701.

Miller BF, et al. 2005. Coordinated collagen and muscle protein synthesis in human patella tendon and quadriceps muscle after exercise. J Physiol 567:1021–1033.

Phillips SM, et al. 1999. Resistance training reduces the acute exercise-induced increase in muscle protein turnover. Am J Physiol Endocrinol Metab 276:E118–E124.

Tipton KD, et al. 1999. Postexercise net protein synthesis in human muscle from orally administered amino acids. Am J Physiol 276:E628–E634.

Biolo G, et al. 1999. Insulin action on muscle protein kinetics and amino acid transport during recovery after resistance exercise. Diabetes 48:949–957.

Churchward-Venne TA, et al. 2012. Nutritional regulation of muscle protein synthesis with resistance exercise: strategies to enhance anabolism. Nutr Metab (London) 9(1):40.

Burd NA, et al. 2010. Resistance exercise volume affects myofibrillar protein synthesis and anabolic signalling molecule phosphorylation in young men. J Physiol 588:3119–3130.

Reitelseder S, et al. 2011. Whey and casein labeled with L-[1-13C]leucine and muscle protein synthesis: effect of resistance exercise and protein ingestion. Am J Physiol Endocrinol Metab. 300:E231–E242.

Symons TB, et al. 2009. A moderate serving of high-quality protein maximally stimulates skeletal muscle protein synthesis in young and elderly subjects. J Am Diet Assoc 109:1582–1586.

Pennings B, et al. 2011. Whey protein stimulates postprandial muscle protein accretion more effectively than do casein and casein hydrolysate in older men. Am J Clin Nutr 93:997–1005.

Wilkinson SB, et al. 2007. Consumption of fluid skim milk promotes greater muscle protein accretion after resistance exercise than does consumption of an isonitrogenous and isoenergetic soy-protein beverage. Am J Clin Nutr 85:1031–1040.

Burd N, et al. 2012. Greater stimulation of myofibrillar protein synthesis with ingestion of whey protein isolate v. micellar casein at rest and after resistance exercise in elderly men. Br J Nutr 108:958–62.

Phillips SM, et al. 2009. The role of milk- and soy-based protein in support of muscle protein synthesis and muscle protein accretion in young and elderly persons. J Am Coll Nutr 28:343–354.

Sharp C, et al. 2010. Amino Acid Supplements and Recovery from High-Intensity Resistance Training. J Strength Cond Res 24(4):1125-1130.

Tipton KD, et al. 1999. Nonessential amino acids are not necessary to stimulate net muscle protein synthesis in healthy volunteers. J Nutr Biochem 10:89–95.

Volpi E, et al. 2003. Essential amino acids are primarily responsible for the amino acid stimulation of muscle protein anabolism in healthy elderly adults. Am J Clin Nutr 78:250–258.

Smith K, et al. 1998. Effects of flooding amino acids on incorporation of labeled amino acids into human muscle protein. Am J Physiol 275:E73–E78.

Anthony JC, et al. 2000. Leucine stimulates translation initiation in skeletal muscle of postabsorptive rats via a rapamycin-sensitive pathway. J Nutr 130:2413–2419.

Crozier SJ, et al. 2005. Oral leucine administration stimulates protein synthesis in rat skeletal muscle. J Nutr 135:376–382.

Atherton PJ, et al. 2010. Distinct anabolic signalling responses to amino acids in C2C12 skeletal muscle cells. Amino Acids 38:1533–1539.

Duan Y, et al. 2015. Nutritional and regulatory roles of leucine in muscle growth and fat reduction. Front Biosci (Landmark Ed) 20:796-813.

Escobar J, et al. 2006. of cardiac and skeletal muscle protein synthesis by individual branched-chain amino acids in neonatal pigs. Am J Physiol Endocrinol Metab 290:E612–E621.

Glynn E, et al. 2010. Excess Leucine Intake Enhances Muscle Anabolic Signaling but Not Net Protein Anabolism in Young Men and Women. J Nutr 140(11):1970-1976.

Conley TB, et al. 2011. Effect of food form on postprandial plasma amino acid concentrations in older adults. Br J Nutr 106:203–207.

Foegeding EA, et al. 2002. Advances in modifying and understanding whey protein functionality. Trend Food Sci Tech 13(5):151-159.

West D, et al. 2011. Rapid aminoacidemia enhances myofibrillar protein synthesis and anabolic intramuscular signaling repsonses after resistance exercise. Am J Clin Nutr 94(3):795–803.

Tang JE, et al. 2009. Ingestion of whey hydrolysate, casein, or soy protein isolate: effects on mixed muscle protein synthesis at rest and following resistance exercise in young men. J Appl Physiol 107(3):987-992.

Boirie Y, et al. 1997. Slow and fast dietary proteins differently modulate postprandial protein accretion. Proc Natl Acad Sci USA 94(26):14930-5.

Yang Y, et al. 2012. Myofibrillar protein synthesis following ingestion of soy protein isolate at rest and after resistance exercise in elderly men. Nutr Metab 9:57.

Mitchell CJ, et al. 2015. Soy protein ingestion results in less prolonged p70s6 kinase phosphorylation compared to whey protein after resistsance exercise in older men. J Inter Soc Sports Nutr 12:6.

Thomson RL, et al. 2015. Muscle strength gains during resistance exercise training are attenuated with soy compared with or usual protein intake in older adults: A randomized controlled trial. Clin Nutr.

Kraemer WJ, et al. 2013. The effects of soy and whey protein supplementation on acute hormonal response resistance exercise in men. J Am Coll Nutr 32(1):66-74.

Acheson KJ, et al. 2011. Protein choices targeting thermogenesis and metabolism. Am J Clin Nutr.

Labayen I, et al. 2004. Basal and postprandial substrate oxidation rates in obese women receiving two test meals with different protein content. Clin Nutr 23:571–8.

Hoffman JR, et al. 2004. Protein – which is best? J Sports Sci Med 3(3):118-130.

Kimball SR, et al. 2006. Signaling pathways and molecular mechanisms through which branched-chain amino acids mediate translational control of protein synthesis. J Nutr 136(1):2275-2315.

Bounous G. 2000. Whey protein concentrate (WPC) and glutathione modulation in cancer treatment. Anticancer Res 20(6C):4785-92.

Fitzpatrick AM, et al. 2012. Glutathione redox control of asthma: from molecular mechanisms to therapeutic opportunities. Antioxid Redox Signal 17(2):3750408.

Chandra RK. 2002. Food hypersensitivity and allergic diseases. Eur J Clin Nutr 56(Suppl 3):S54-6.

Loss G, et al. 2011. The protective effect of farm milk consumption on childhood asthma and atopy: the GABRIELA study. J Allergy Clin Immunol 128(4):766-773.

Markus CR, et al. Whey protein rich in alpha-lactalbumin increases the ratio of plasma tryptophan to the sum of the other large neutral amino acids and improves cognitive performance in stress-vulnerable subjects. Am J Clin Nutr 75(6):1051-6.

Said HM, et al. 1989. Intestinal uptake of retinol: enhancement by bovine milk beta-lactoglobulin. Am J Clin Nutr 49(4):690-4.

Sprong RC, et al. 2010. Dietary cheese whey protein protects rats against dextra sulphate sodium-induced colitis mucin and microbiota. J Dairy Sci 93(4):1364-71.

Shertzer HG, et al. 2013. Dietary whey protein stimulates mitochondrial activity and decreases oxidative stress in mouse brain. Neurosci Lett 548:159-64.

Benjamin J, et al. 2012. Glutamin and whey protein improve intestinal permeability and morphology in patients with disease: a randomized controlled trial. Dig Dis Sci 57(4):1000-12.

Bruck WM, et al. 2014. The effect of proteolysis on the induction of cell death by monomeric alpha-lactalbumin. Biochimie 97:138-43.

Rodrigues L, et al. 2009. Lactoferrin and cancer disease prevention. Crit Rev Food Sci Nutr 49(3):203-17.

Kanwar RK, et al. 2013. Immunomodulatory lactoferrin in the regulation of apoptosis modulatory proteins in cancer. Protein Pept Lett 20(4):450-8.

Bortolotti M, et al. 2011. Effects of a whey protein supplementation on intrahepatocellular lipids in obese female patients. Clin Nutr 30(4):494-8.

Chitapanarux T, et al. 2009. Open-labeled pilot study of cysteine-rich whey protein isolate supplementation for non-alcoholic steatohepatitis patients. J Gastroenterol Hepatol 24(6):1045-50.

Wlodarski KH, et al. 2014. The importance of lactoferrin in bone regeneration. Pol Merkur Lekarski 37(217):65-7.

Delmi M, et al. 1990. Dietary Supplementation in Elderly Patients with Fractured Neck of the Femur. Lancet 355(1990):1013-1016.

Aoe S, et al. 2001. Controlled trial of the effects of milk basic protein (MBP) supplementation on bone metabolism healthy adult women. Biosci Biotechnol Biochem 65(4):913-8.

Hall WL, et al. 2003. Casein and whey exert different effects on plasma amino acid profiles, gastrointestinal hormone secretion and appetite. Br J Nutr 89(2):239-48.

Hursel R, et al. 2010. Effects of a breakfast yoghurt, with additional total whey protein or caseinomacropeptide-depleted alpha-lactalbumin-enriched whey protein, or diet-induced thermogenesis and appetite suppression. Br J Nutr 103(5):775-80.

Pal S, et al. 2010. Effects of whey protein isolate on body composition, lipids, insulin and glucose in overweight and obese individuals. Br J Nutr 104(5):716-23.

Madzima TA, et al. 2014. Night-time consumption of protein or carbohydrate results in increased morning resting energy expenditure in active college-aged men. Br J Nutr 111(1):71-7.

FitzGerald RJ, et al. 2004. Hypotensive peptides from milk proteins. J Nutr 134(4):980S-8S.

Pal S, et al. 2013. The effects of whey protein on cardiometabolic risk factors. Obes Rev 14(4):324-43.

Marshall K. 2004. Therapeutic applications of whey protein. Altern Med Rev 9(2):136-56.

Bounous G, et al. 1991. Whey proteins in cancer prevention. Cancer Lett 57(2):91-4.

Kent KD, et al. Effect of whey protein isolate on intracellular glutathione and oxidant-induced cell death in human prostate epithelial cells. Toxicol in Vitro 17(1):27-33.

McIntosh GH. 1993. Colon cancer: dietary modifications required for a balanced protective diet. Prev Med 22(5):767-74.

Hakkak R, et al. 2001. Dietary Whey Protein Protects against Azoxymethane-Induced Colon Tumors in Male Rats. Cancer Epidem Biom Preve 10 (5):555-558.

Appleton BS, et al. 1982. Inhibition of aflatoxin-initiated preneoplastic liver lesions by low dietary protein. Nutr Cancer 3(4):200-6.

Appleton BS, et al. 1983. Effect of high and low dietary protein on the dosing and postdosing periods of aflatoxin B1-induced hepatic preneoplastic lesion development in the rat. Cancer Res 43(5):2150-4.

Power O, et al. 2009. Human insulinotropic response to oral ingestion of native and hydrolysed whey protein. Amino Acids 37(2):333-9.

Bounous G, et al. 1991. The biological activity of undenatured dietary whey proteins: role of glutathione. Clin Invest Med 14(4):296-309.

Douglas FW Jr., et al. 1981. Effect of ultra-high-temperature pasteurization on milk proteins. J Agric Food Chem 29(1):11-15.

Sheikholeslami VD, et al. 2012. Changes in antioxidant status and cardiovascular risk factors of overweight young men after six weeks supplementation of whey protein isolate and resistance training. Appetite 59(3):673-8.

Mitchell WK, et al. 2014. A dose- rather than delivery profile- dependent mechanism regulates the "muscle-full" effect in response to oral essential amino acid intake in young men. J Nutr 114:199604.

Moore DR, et al. 2009. Ingested protein dose response of muscle and albumin protein synthesis after resistance exercise in young men. Am J Clin Nutr 89:161–168.

Witard O, et al. 2014. Myofibrillar muscle protein synthesis rates subsequent to a meal in response to increasing doses of whey protein at rest and after resistance exercise. Am J Clin Nutr 99(1):86–95.

Hulmi J, et al. 2010. Effect of Protein/Essential Amino Acids and Resistance Training on Skeletal Muscle Hypertrophy. Nutr Metab 7(51).

Areta JL, et al. 2014. Increasing leucine concentration stimulates mechanistic target of rapamycin signaling and cell growth in C2C12 skeletal muscle cells. Nutr Res 34(11):1000-7.

Churchward-Venne TA, et al. 2014. Leucine supplementation of a low-protein mixed macronutrient beverage enhances myofibrillar protein synthesis in young men: a double-blind, randomized trial. Am J Clin Nutr 99(2):276-286.

Tipton KD, et al. 2009. Stimulation of muscle anabolism by resistance exercise and ingestion of leucine plus protein. Appl Phys 34:151–161.

Baumgartner RN, et al. 1998. Epidemiology of sarcopenia among the elderly in New Mexico. Am J Epidemiol 147:755–763.

Raguso CA, et al. 2006. A 3-year longitudinal study on body composition changes in the elderly: role of physical exercise. Clin Nutr 25:573–580.

Kumar V, et al. 2009. Age-related differences in the dose–response relationship of muscle protein synthesis to resistance exercise in young and old men. J Physiol 587:211–217.

Cuthbertson D, et al. 2005. Anabolic signaling deficits underlie amino acid resistance of wasting, aging muscle. FASEB J 19:422–424.

Breen L, et al. 2012. Interactions between exercise and nutrition to prevent muscle waste during aging. Br J Clin Pharmacol.

Sheffield-Moore M, et al. 2005. Mixed muscle and hepatic derived plasma protein metabolism is differentially regulated in older and younger men following resistance exercise. Am J Physiol Endocrinol Metab 288:E922–E929.

Volpi E, et al. 2000. The response of muscle protein anabolism to combined hyperaminoacidemia and glucose-induced hyperinsulinemia is impaired in the elderly. J Clin Endocrinol Metab 85:4481–4490.

Drummond MJ, et al. 2008. Skeletal muscle protein anabolic response to resistance exercise and essential amino acids is delayed with aging. J Appl Physiol 104:1452–1461.

Symons TB, et al. 2011. The anabolic response to resistance exercise and a protein-rich meal is not diminished by age. J Nutr Health Aging 15:376–381.

Doherty TJ. Invited review: Aging and sarcopenia. J Appl Physiol 95:1717–1727

Yang Y, et al. 2012. Resistance exercise enhances myofibrillar protein synthesis with graded intakes of whey protein in older men. Br J Nutr.

Masterjohn, Chris. "With the Wave of a Wand, Raw Milk Wipes Away the Wheeze: How Our Good Friend Glutathione Protects Against Asthma." Weston A Price. Mar. 2012.

Carbonaro M, et al. 1997. Disulfide reactivity and in vitro protein digestability of different thermal-treated milk samples and whey proteins. J Agric Food Chem 45(1):95-100.

Volek JS, et al. 2013. Whey protein supplementation during resistance training augments lean body mass. J Am Coll Nutr 32(2):122-35.

Dreyer HC, et al. 2008. Leucine-enriched essential amino acid and carbohydrate ingestion following resistance exercise enhances mTOR signaling and protein synthesis in human muscle. Am J Physiol Endocrinol Metab 294:E392–E400.

Borsheim E, et al. 2004 Effect of an amino acid, protein, and carbohydrate mixture on net muscle protein balance after resistance exercise. Int J Sport Nutr Exerc Metab 14:255–271.

Borsheim E, et al. 2004. Effect of carbohydrate intake on net muscle protein synthesis during recovery from resistance exercise. J Appl Physiol 96:674–678.

Borsheim E, et al. 2002. Essential amino acids and muscle protein recovery from resistance exercise. Am J Physiol Endocrinol Metab 283:E648–E657.

Fujita S, et al. 2007. Nutrient signalling in the regulation of human muscle protein synthesis. J Physiol 582:813–823.

Dickinson JM, et al. 2014. Leucine-enriched amino acid ingestion after resistance exercise prolonges myofibrillar protein synthesis and amino acid transporter expression in older men. J Nutr 144(11):1694-702.

Bukhari, et al. 2015. Intake of low-dose leucine-rich essential amino acids stimulates muscle anabolism equivalently to bolus whey protein in older women at rest. Am J Physiol Endocr Metab 308(12):E1056-E1065.

Hawley JA, et al. 2011. Nutritional modulation of training-induced skeletal muscle adaptations. J Appl Physiol 110(3):834-845.

Katsanos CS, et al. 2006. A high proportion of leucine is required for optimal stimulation of the rate of muscle protein synthesis by essential amino acids in the elderly. Am J Physiol Endocrinol Metab 291:E381–E387.

Anthony J, et al. 2001. Signalling pathways involved in translational control of protein synthesis in skeletal muscle by leucine. J Nutr 131:856S–60S.

Baer DJ, et al. 2011. Whey protein but not soy protein supplementation alters body weight and composition in free-living overweight and obese adults. J Nutr 141(8):1489-94.

Katsanos CS, et al. Muscle protein synthesis and balance responsiveness to essential amino acids ingestion in the presence of elevated plasma free fatty acid concentrations. J Clin Endocrinol Metab 94(8):2984-90.

Fox AK, et al. 2004. Adding fat calories to meals after exercise does not alter glucose tolerance. J Appl Physiol 97(1):11-6.

Miller PE, et al. 2014. Effects of whey protein and resistance exercise on body composition: a meta-analysis of randomized controlled trials. J Am Coll Nutr 33(2):163-75.

Arciero PJ, et al. Timed-daily ingestion of whey protein and exercise training reduces visceral adipose tissue mass and improves insulin resistance: the PRISE study. J Appl Physiol.

Phillips BE, et al. Regulation of muscle protein synthesis in humans. Curr Opin Nutr Metab Care 15(1):58-63.

Glynn EL, et al. 2013. Addition of carbohydrate or alanine to an essential amino acid mixture does not enhance human skeletal muscle protein anabolism. J Nutr 143(3):307-314.

Slater G, et al. 2011. Nutrition guidelines for strength sports: sprinting, weightlifting, throwing events, and bodybuilding. J Sports Sci 29(1):S67–77.

Camera DM, et al. 2012. Low muscle glycogen concentration does not suppress the anabolic response to resistance exercise. J Apply Physiol (1985) 113(2):206-14.

Kerksick C, et al. 2008. International Society of Sports Nutrition position stand: nutrient timing. J Int Soc Sports Nutr 5:17.

Staples AW, et al. 2011. Carbohydrate does not augment exercise-induced protein accretion versus protein alone. Med Sci Sports Exerc 43:1154–1161.

Iverson JF, et al. 2014. Interaction of ingested leucine with glycine on insulin and glucose concentrations. J Amino Acids 2014:521941.

Trommelen J, et al. 2015. Exogenous insulin does not increase muscle protein synthesis rate when administrated systemically: a systematic review. Eur J Endocr 14:0902.

Trombold JR, et al. 2014. Postexercise macronutrient intake and subsequent postprandial triglyceride metabolism. Med Sci Sports Exerc.

Gelfand RA, et al. 1987. Effect of physiologic hyperinsulinemia on skeletal muscle protein synthesis and breakdown in man. J Clin Invest 80:1–6.

Denne SC, et al. 1991. Proteolysis in skeletal muscle and whole body in response to euglycemic hyperinsulinemia in normal adults. Am J Physiol 261(6 Pt 1):E809-14.

Heslin MJ, et al. 1992. Effect of hyperinsulinemia on whole body and skeletal muscle leucine carbon kinetics in humans. Am J Physiol 262(6 Pt 1):E911-8.

Kettelhut IC, et al. 1988. Endocrine regulation of protein breakdown in skeletal muscle. Diabetes Metab Rev 4(8):751-72.

Biolo G, et al. 1997. An abundant supply of amino acids enhances the metabolic effect of exercise on muscle protein. Am J Physiol 273(1 Pt 1):E122-9.

Glynn EL, et al. 2010. Muscle protein breakdown has a minor role in the protein anabolic response to essential amino acid and carbohydrate intake following resistance exercise. Am J Physiol Regul Integr Comp Physiol 299(2):R533-40.

Floyd JC Jr, et al. 1963. Evidence that insulin release is the mechanism for experimentally induced leucine hypoglycemia in man. J Clin Invest 42:1714–1719.

Anthony JC, et al. 2002. Contribution of insulin to the translational control of protein synthesis in skeletal muscle by leucine. Am J Physiol Endocrinol Metab 282(5):E1092–1101.

Hamer HM, et al. 2013. Carbohydrate co-ingestion with protein does not further augment post-prandial muscle protein accretion in older men. Nutr Metab (Lond) 10(1):15.

Miller SL, et al. 2003. Independent and combined effects of amino acids and glucose after resistance exercise. Medicine and science in sports and exercise. 35:449–455.

Greenhaff PL, et al. 2008. Disassociation between the effects of amino acids and insulin on signaling, ubiquitin ligases, and protein turnover in human muscle. Am J Physiol Endocrinol Metab 295:E595–E604.

Zawadzki KM, et al. 1992. Carbohydrate-protein complex increases the rate of muscl glycogen storage after exercise. J Appl Physiol 72(5):1854-1859.

Robergs RA, et al. 1991. Muscle glycogenolysis during differing intensities of weight-resistance exercise. J Appl Physiol 70(4):1700-6.

Roy BD, et al. 1998. Influence of differing macronutrient intakes on muscle glycogen resynthesis after resistance exercise. J Appl Physiol 84(3):890-6.

Figueiredo VC, et al. 2013. Is carbohydrate needed to further stimulate muscle protein synthesis/hypertrophy following resistance exercise? J Int Soc Sports Nutr 10:42.

Koopman R, et al. 2007. Coingestion of carbohydrate with protein does not further augment postexercise muscle protein synthesis. Am J Physiol Endocrinol Metab 293(3):E833-42.

Pascoe DD, et al. 1993. Glycogen resynthesis in skeletal muscle following resistive exercise. Med Sci Sports Exerc1925:349–354

Jakubowics D, et al. 2012. Biochemical and Metabolic Mechanisms by Which Dietary Whey Protein May Combat Obesity and Type 2 Diabetes. J Nutri Biochem.

Kim M, et al. 2015. The combination of ursolic acid and leucine potentiates the differentiation of C2C12 murine myoblasts through the mTOR signalling pathway. Int J Mol Med 35(3):755-62.

Tipton KD, et al. 2001. Timing of amino acid-carbohydrate ingestion alters anabolic response of muscle to resistance exercise. Am J Physiol Endocrinol Metab 281(2):E197-206.

Ivy J, et al. 2004. Nutrient timing: The future of sports nutrition. North Bergen, NJ: Basic Health Publications.

Cribb PJ, et al. 2006. Effects of supplement timing and resistance exercise on skeletal muscle hypertrophy. Med Sci Sports Exerc 38(11):1918-1925.

Willoughby DS, et al. 2007. Effects of resistance training and protein plus amino acid supplementation on muscle anabolism, mass, and strength. Amino Acids 32(4):467-477.

Hulmi JJ, et al. 2009. Acute and long-term effects of resistance exercise with or without protein ingestion on muscle hypertrophy and gene expression. Amino Acids 37(2):297-308.

Burk A, et al. 2009. Time-divided ingestion pattern of casein-based protein supplement stimulates an increase in fat-free body mass during resistance training in young untrained men. Nutr Res 29(6):405-413.

Esmarck B, et al. 2001. Timing of postexercise protein intake is important for muscle hypertrophy with resistance training in elderly humans. J Physiol 535(Pt 1):301-11.

Lemon PW, et al. 2002. The role of protein and amino acid supplements in the athlete's diet: does type or timing of ingestion matter? Curr Sports Med Rep 1(4):214-221.

Aragon AA, et al. 2013. Nutrient timing revisited: is there a post-exercise anabolic window? J Int Soc Sports Nutr 10(1):10-15.

Schoenfeld BJ, et al. The effect of protein timing on muscle strength and hypertrophy: a meta-analysis. J Inter Soc Sports Nutr 10:53.

Kumar V, et al. 2009. Human muscle protein synthesis and breakdown during and after exercise. J Appl Physiol 106(6):2026-39.

Atherton PJ, et al. 2010. Muscle full effect after oral protein: time-dependent concordance and discordance between human muscle protein synthesis and mTORC1 signaling. Am J Clin Nutr 92(5):1080-8.

Bohe J, et al. 2001. Latency and duration of stimulation of human muscle protein synthesis during continuous infusion of amino acids. J Physiol 2001, 532(Pt 2):575-9.

Pitkanen HT, et al. 2003. Free amino acid pool and muscle protein balance after resistance exercise. Med Sci Sports Exerc 35(5):784-92.

Ivy JL. 1998. Glycogen resynthesis after exercise: effect of carbohydrate intake. Int J Sports Med. 19(Suppl 2):S142-5.

Parkin JA, et al. 1997. Muscle glycogen storage following prolonged exercise: effect of timing of ingestion of high glycemic index food. Med Sci Sports Exerc 29(2):220-4.

Rasmussen BB, et al. 2000. An oral essential amino-acid carbohydrate supplement enhances muscle protein anabolism after resistance exercise. J Appl Physiol (1985) 88(2):386-92.

Witard OC, et al. 2014. Increased net muscle protein balance in response to simultaneous and separate ingestion of carbohydrate and essential amino acids following resistance exercise. Appl Physol Nutr Metab 39(3):329-39.

Chtourou H, et al. 2012. The effect of strength training at the same time of day on the diurnal fluctuations of muscular anaerobic performances. J Strength Cond Res 26(1):217-25.

Principle #9

Paffenbarger RS, et al. 2004. The “weekend warrior” and risk of mortality. Am J Epidem 160(7):636-41.

Bobbert MA, et al. 1994. Effects of muscle strengthening on vertical jump height: a simulation study. Med Sci Sports Exerc 26:1012-20.

Daskalopoulou SS, et al. 2014. Plasma irisin levels progressively increase in response to increasing exercise workloads in young, healthy, active subjects. Eur J Endocrinol 171(3):343-52.

Trapp EG, et al. 2008. The effects of high-intensity intermittent exercise training on fat loss and fasting insulin levels of young women. Int J Obes 32(4):684-691.

Tremblay A, et al. 1994. Impact of exercise intensity on body fatness and skeletal muscle metabolism. Metabolism 43:814–818.

Bahr R, et al. 1992. Effect of intensity of exercise on excess postexercise O 2 consumption. Metabolism 40:836–841.

Paoli A, et al. 2012. High-Intensity Interval Resistance Training Influences Resting Energy Expenditure and Respiratory Ratio in Non-Dieting Individuals. J Trans Med 10(1):237.

Volek JS, et al. 1997. Testosterone and cortisol in relationship to dietary nutrients and resistance exercise. J Appl Physiol 82(1):49-54.

Barres R, et al. 2012. Acute exercise remodels promoter methylation in human skeletal muscle. Cell Metab 15(3):405-411.

Sakharov D, et al. 2011. Passing the Anaerobic Threshold is Associated with Substantial Changes in eh Gene Expression Profile in White Blood Cells. Eur J Appl Physiol.

Godfrey RJ, et al. 2003. The exercise-induced growth hormone response in athletes. Sports Med 33(8):599-613.

Wideman L, et al. 2002. Growth hormone release during acute and chronic aerobic and resistance exercise: recent findings. Sports Med 32(15):987-1004.

Sutton J, et al. 1976. Growth hormone in exercise: comparison of physiological and pharmacological stimuli. J Appl Physiol 41:523-27.

Kraemer WJ, et al. 2005. Hormonal responses and adaptations to resistance exercise and training. Sport Med 35:339–361.

Iida K, et al. 2004. Muscle mechano growth factor is preferentially induced by growth hormone in growth hormonedeficient lit/lit mice. J Physiol 15(560):341–349.

Hameed M, et al. 2004. The effect of recombinant human growth hormone and resistance training on IGF-I mRNA expression in the muscles of elderly men. J Physiol 555: 231–240.

Barton-Davis, ER, Shoturma, DI, and Sweeney, HL. Contribution of satellite cells to IGF-I induced hypertrophy of skeletal muscle. Acta Physiol Scan 167: 301–305, 1999.

Hill M, et al. 2003. Expression and splicing of the insulinlike growth factor gene in rodent muscle is associated with muscle satellite (stem) cell activation following local tissue damage. J Physiol 549:409–418.

Yang SY, et al. 2002. Different roles of the IGF-IEc peptide (MGF) and mature IGF-I in myoblast proliferation and differentiation. FEBS Lett 522:156–160.

Musaro A, et al. 1999. IGF-1 induces skeletal myocyte hypertrophy through calcineurin in association with GATA-2 and NF-ATc1. Nature 400:581–585.

Janssen I, et al. 2012. Vigorous intensity physical activity is related to the metabolic syndrome independent of the physical activity dose. Int J Epidem 41(4):1132–1140.

Buchheit M, et al. 2013. High-intensity interval training, solutions to the programming puzzle: part I: cardiopulmonary emphasis. Sports Med. 43:313-338.

Kemi OJ, et al. 2005. Moderate vs. high exercise intensity: Differential effects on aerobic fitness, cardiomyocyte contractility, and endothelial function. Cardiovasc Res 67:161-172.

Wisløff U, et al. 2007. Superior cardiovascular effect of aerobic interval training versus moderate continuous training in heart failure patients: A randomized study. Circulation 115:3086– 3094.

Rognmo O, et al. 2012. Cardiovascular risk of high- versus moderate-intensity aerobic exercise in coronary heart disease patients. Circulation 126(12):1436-1440.

Rakobowchuk MS, et al. 2008. Sprint interval and traditional endurance training induce similar improvements in peripheral arterial stiffness and flow-mediated dilation in healthy humans. Am J Physiol 295:R236-R242.

Ramos JS, et al. 2015. The impact of high-intensity interval training versus moderate-intensity continuous training on vascular function: a systematic review and meta-analysis. Sports Med 45(5):679-692.

Matsuo T, et al. 2014. Effects of a low-volume aerobic-type interval exercise on VO_2max and cardiac mass. Med Sci Sports Exerc 46:42-50.

Matsuo T, et al. 2015. Low-volume, high-intensity, aerobic interval exercise for sedentary adults: vo2max, cardiac mass, and heart rate recovery. Eur J Appl Physiol 114(9):1963-72.

Cocks M, et al. 2013. Sprint interval and endurance training are equally effective in increasing muscle microvascular density and eNOS content in sedentary males. J Physiol 591:641-656.

Tjønna AE, et al. 2008. Aerobic interval training versus continuous moderate exercise as a treatment for the metabolic syndrome: A pilot study. Circulation 118:346–354.

Hallmark R, et al. 2014. The effect of exercise on endothelial function in physically inactive lean and obese adults. PLoS ONE 9(1):e85450.

Klonizakis M, et al. 2014. Low-volume high-intensity interval training rapidly improves cardiopulmonary function in postmenopausal women. Menopause 21(10):1099-105.

Neunteufl T, et al. 2000. Late prognostic value of flow-mediated dilation in the brachial artery of patients with chest pain. Am J Cardiol 86:207–210.

Green DJ, et al. 2004. Effect of exercise training on endothelium-derived nitric oxide function in humans. J Physiol 561:1–25.

Celermajer DS, et al. 1994. Endothelium-dependent dilation in the systemic arteries of asymptomatic subjects relates to coronary risk factors and their interaction. J Am Coll Cardiol 24:1468–1474.

Wisløff U, et al. 2009. High-intensity interval training to maximize cardiac benefits of exercise training? Exerc Sport Sci Rev 37(3):139–146.

Tjønna AE, et al. 2009. Aerobic interval training reduces cardiovascular risk factors more than a multitreatment approach in overweight adolescents. Clinical Science 116(4):317-326.

Ma JK, et al. 2013. Extremely low-volume, high-intensity interval training improves exercise capacity and increases mitochondrial protein content in human skeletal muscle. J Mol Integr Physiol 3:202–210.

Gillen JB, et al. 2014. Three minutes of all-out intermittent exercise per week increases skeletal muscle oxidative capacity and improves cardiometabolic health. 9(11):e111489.

Metcalfe RS, et al. 2011. Towards the minimal amount of exercise for improving metabolic health: beneficial effects of reduced-exertion high-intensity interval training. Eur J Appl Physiol 112:2767–2775.

Racil G, et al. 2013. Effects of high vs. moderate exercise intensity during interval training on lipids and adiponectin levels in obese young females. Eur J Appl Physiol 113(1):2531-40.

Deus A, et al. 2011. Metabolic and Cardiac Autonomic Effects of High-Intensity Resistance Training Protocol in Wistar Rats. J Strength Cond Res.

Ortega JF, et al. 2015. Higher Insulin-sensitizing response after sprint interval compared to continuous exercise. 36(03):209-214.

Burgomaster KA, et al. 2006. Effect of short-term sprint interval training on human skeletal muscle carbohydrate metabolism during exercise and time-trial performance. J Appl Physiol 100(6):2041-7.

Sandvei M, et al. 2012. Sprint interval running increases insulin sensitivity in young healthy subjects. Arch Physiol Biochem 118(3):139-47.

Whyte LJ, et al. 2010. Effect of 2 weeks of sprint interval training on health-related outcomes in sedentary overweight/obese men. Metabolism 59(10):1421-8.

Babraj JA, et al. 2009. Extremely short duration high intensity interval training substantially improves insulin action in young healthy males. BMC Endocr Disord 9:3.

Freese EC, et al. 2011. Effects of acute sprint interval cycling and energy replacement on postprandial lipemia. J Appl Physiol 111(6):1584-9.

Richards JC, et al. 2010. Short-term sprint interval training increases insulin sensitivity in healthy adults but does not affect the thermogenic response to beta-adrenergic stimulation. J Physiol 588:2961–2972.

Freese EC, et al. 2015. Acute and chronic effects of sprint interval exercise on postprandial lipemia in women at risk for the metabolic syndrome. J Appl Physiol

Akasaki Y, et al. 2014. Glycolytic fast-twich muscle fiber restoration counters adverse age-related changes in body composition and metabolism. Aging Cell 13(1):80-91.

Walker S, et al. 2015. Medium-intensity, high-volume 'hypertrophic' resistance training did not induce improvements in rapid force production in healthy older men. Age (Dordr) 37(3):9786.

Burgomaster KA, et al. 2005. Six sessions of sprint interval training increases muscle oxidative potential and cycle endurance capacity. J Appl Physiol 98:1895-1990.

Gibala MJ, et al. 2006. Short-term sprint interval versus traditional endurance training: similar initial adaptations in human skeletal muscle and exercise performance. J Physiol 575:901-911.

Saltin B, and Gollnick PD. 1983. Skeletal muscle adaptability: significance for metabolism and performance. In L.D. Peachey (ed.) Handbook of Physiology. Skeletal Muscle. pp. 555-631, American Physiological Society, Bethesda.

Little JP, et al. 2010. A practical model of low-volume high-intensity interval training induces mitochondrial biogenesis in human skeletal muscle: potential mechanisms. J Physiol 586:1011-1022.

Hood MS, et al. 2011. Low-Volume Interval Training Improves Muscle Oxidative Capacity in Sedentary Adults. Med Sci Sports Exerc 43:1849–1856.

Kubukeli ZN, et al. 2002. Training techniques to improve endurance exercise performances. Sports Med. 32:489-509.

Ross A, et al. 2001. Long-term metabolic and skeletal muscle adaptations to short-sprint training: implications for sprint training and tapering. Sports Med 31:1063-1082.

Kodama S, et al. 2009. Cardiorespiratory fitness as a quantitative predictor of all-cause mortality and cardiovascular events in healthy men and women: a meta-analysis. JAMA 301(19):2024-2035.

Fleck SJ. 1988. Cardiovascular adaptations to resistance training. Med Sci Sports Exerc. 20:S146-51.

Porter C, et al. 2014. Resistance exercise training alters mitochondrial function in Human Skeletal Muscle. Med Sci Sports Exerc.

Moholdt T, et al. 2014. The higher the better? Interval training intensity in coronary heart disease. J Science Med Sport 17(5):506-510.

Gibala MJ, et al. 2014. Physiological and health-related adaptations to low-volume interval training: influences of nutrition and sex. Sports Med. 44 Suppl 2:127-137.

Dudley G, et al. 1982. Influence of exercise intensity and duration on biochemical adaptations in skeletal muscle. J Appl Physiol 53:844-50.

Davies C, et al. 1971. The training stimulus: The effects of intensity, duration, and frequency of effort on maximum aerobic power output. Int. 2. Angew: 20:299-305.

Gibala MJ, et al. 2009. Brief intense interval exercise activates AMPK and p38 MAPK signaling and increases the expression of PGC-1α in human skeletal muscle. J Appl Physiol 106:929-934.

Little JP, et al. 2011. An acute bout of high-intensity interval training increases the nuclear abundance of PGC- 1α and activates mitochondrial biogenesis in human skeletal muscle. Am J Physiol 300:R1303-1310.

Burgomaster KA, et al. 2008. Similar metabolic adaptations during exercise after low volume sprint interval and traditional endurance training in humans. J Physiol 586:151-160.

Perry CG, et al. 2010. Repeated transient mRNA bursts precede increases in transcriptional and mitochondrial proteins during training in human skeletal muscle. J. Physiol 588:4795-4810.

MacDougall JD, et al. 1998. Muscle performance and enzymatic adaptations to sprint interval training. J Appl Physiol 84:2138-2142.

Jacobs AR, et al. 2013. Improvements in exercise performance with high-intensity interval training coincide with an increase in skeletal muscle mitochondrial content and function. J Appl Physiol 115(6):785-793.

Vincent G, et al. 2015. Changes in mitochondrial function and mitochondria associated protein expression in response to 2-weeks in high intensity interval training. Front Physiol 6:51.

Weston KS, et al. 2014. High-intensity interval training in patients with lifestyle-induced cardiometabolic disease: a systematic review and meta-analysis. Br J Sports Med 48:1227-1234.

Koli J, et al. 2005. Effect of Exercise on Patellar Cartilage in Women with Mild Knee Osteoarthritis. Medicine & Science in Sports & Exercise.

Mero AMJ. 2014. Effects of power versus endurance training on bone metabolism markers, serum hormone concentrations and physical performance in young athletes. University of Jyväskylä.

Haakinen K, et al. 1985. Changes in electrical and mechanical behavior of leg extensor muscles during heavy resistance strength training. Scand J Sports Sci 7:55-64.

Haakinen K, et al. 1985. The effect of explosive type strength training on electromyographic and force production characteristics of leg extensor muscle during concentric and various stretch-shortening cycle exercises. Scand J Sports Sci 7:65-76.

Macpherson R, et al. 2011. Run Sprint Interval Training Improves Aerobic Performance but Not Maximal Cardiac Output. Med Sci Sports Exerc 43(1):115-121.

Cauthon DJ, et al. 2012. Minimalist shoe injuries: Three case reports. Int J Clin Foot Science 23(203):100-103.

Robbins S, et al. 1993. Protective sensation of the plantar aspect of the foot. Foot and Ankle 14:347-352

Olin ED, et al. 2013. EMG and tibial shock upon the first attempt at barefoot running. Human Mov Sci 32(2):343-52.

Lieberman DE, et al. 2010. Foot strike patterns and collision forces in habitually barefoot versus shod runners. Nature 463:531-535.

Peri DP, et al. 2012. Effects of footwear and strike type on running economy. Med Sci Sports Exerc 44(7):1335-43.

Kulmala JP, et al. 2013. Forefoot strikers exhibit lower running-induced knee loading than rearfoot strikers. Med Sci Sports Exerc 45(12):2306-13.

Bonacci J, et al. 2013. Take your shoes off to reduce patellofemoral joint stress during running. Br J Sports Med.

Bergmann G, et al. 1995. Influence of shoes and heel strike on the loading of the hip joint. J Biomech 28:817-827.

Diebal AR, et al. 2011. Effects of forefoot running on chronic exertional compartment syndrome: a case series. Int J Sports Phys Ther 6(4):312-21.

Diebal AR, et al. 2012. Forefoot running improves pain and disability associated with exertional compartment syndrome. 40(5):1060-7.

Frederick EC. 1986. Kinematically mediated effects of sports shoe design: a review. J Sport Sci 4:169-184

Siff MC and Verkhoshansky YV. 1999. Supertraining (4th ed.). Denver, Colorado. Supertraining International.

Yessis M (2000). Explosive running. Illinois, USA. Contemporary Books.

Robbins SE, et al. 1995. Ankle taping improves proprioception before and after exercise in young men. Br J Sport Med 29:242-247.

Stacoff A, et al. 1996. Lateral stability in sideward cutting movements. Med Sci Sport Exerc 28:350-358.

Robbins SE, et al. 1987. Running-related injury prevention through barefoot adaptations. Med Sci Sport Exerc 19:148-156.

Robbins SE, et al. 1989. Running-related injury prevention through innate impact-moderating behavior. Med Sci Sport Exerc 21:130-139.

Robbins SE, et al. 1990. Athletic footwear and chronic overloading: a brief review. Sport Med 9:76-85.

Wegener C, et al. 2011. Effect of children's shoes on gait: a systematic review and meta-analysis. J Foot Ankle Res 4:3.

Wilson GJ, et al. 1993. The optimal training load for the development of dynamic athletic performance. Med Sci Sports Exerc 25:1279-86.

Lake JP, et al. 2012. Kettlebell swing improves maximal and explosive strength. J Strength Cond Res 26(8):2228-33.

Wilson, GJ, et al. 1997. Performance benefits from weight and plyometric training: Effects of initial strength level. Coach Sport Sci J 2:3-8.

Ebben W, et al. Magnitude and Rate of Mechanical Loading of a Variety of Exercise Modes. J Strength Cond Res 24(1):213-217.

Parolin ML, et al. 1999. Regulation of skeletal muscle glycogen phosphorylase and PDH during maximal intermittent exercise. Am J Physiol 277:E890-900.

Hazell TJ, et al. 2010. 10 or 30-S Sprint Interval Training Bouts Enhance Both Aerobic and Anaerobic Performance. Eur J Appl Physiol 110:153–160.

Blair SN, Brodney S (1999) Effects of physical inactivity and obesity on morbidity and mortality: current evidence and research issues. Med Sci Sports Exerc 31:S646–62.

Stathokostas L, et al. 2004. Longitudinal changes in aerobic power in older men and women. J Appl Physiol 97(2):781–9.

Tabata I, et al. 1996. Effects of moderate-intensity endurance and high-intensity intermittent training on anaerobic capacity and VO2max. Med Sci Sports Exerc 28:1327–1330.

Tjønna AE, et al. Low- and high-volume of intensive endurance training significantly improves maximal oxygen uptake after 10-weeks of training in healthy men. PLoS One 8:e65382.

Murach K, et al. Is Long Duration Aerobic Exercise Necessary For Anaerobic Athletes. Strength Cond J 35(2), 44-46.

Wilson et al. 2012. Concurrent Training: a Meta-Analysis Examining Interference of Aerobic and Resistance Exercises. J Strength Cond Res 26(8):2293-2307.

Ronnestad B, et al. 2012. High Volume of Endurance Training Impairs Adaptations to 12 Weeks of Strength Training in Well-Trained Endurance Athletes. Eur J Appl Physiol 112:1457-1466.

Larose J, et al. 2011. Comparison of Strength Development with Resistance Training and combined Exercise Training in Type 2 Diabetes. Scan J Med Sci Sport.

Cantrelli et al. 2014. Maximal strength, power, and aerobic endurance adaptations to concurrent strength and sprint interval training. Eur J Apply Physiol 114:763-771.

Vogel T, et al. 2009. Health benefits of physical activity in older patients: a review. Int J Clin Prac 63(2):303–20.

Kessler HS, et al. 2012. The potential for high-intensity interval training to reduce cardiometabolic disease risk. Sports Med 42:489-509.

Little JP, et al. 2011. Low-volume high- intensity interval training reduces hyperglycemia and increases muscle mitochondrial capacity in patients with type 2 diabetes. J Appl Physiol 111(6):1554–1560.

Rynders CA, et al. 2014. High-intensity exercise training for the prevention of type 2 diabetes mellitus. Physic Sports Med 42:1.

Gayda M, et al. 2012. Central hemodynamic responses during acute high-intensity interval exercise and moderate continuous exercise in patients with heart failure. Appl Physiol Nutr Metab 37(6):1171-1178.

Gillen JP, et al. 2012. Acute high-intensity interval exercise reduces the postprandial glucose response and prevalence of hyperglycaemia in patients with type 2 diabetes. Diab Obes Metab 14(6):575-577.

Francois ME, et al. 2014. Exercise snacks' before meals: a novel strategy to improve glycaemic control in individuals with insulin resistance. Diabetologia 57(7):1437-1445.

Karstoft K, et al. 2012. The effects of free-living interval-walking training on glycemic control, body composition, and physical fitness in type 2 diabetic patients: a randomized, controlled trial. Diabetes Care 36(2):228-236.

Trost SG, et al. 2002. Correlates of adults' participation in physical activity: review and update. Med Science Sport Exerc 34(12):1996-2001.

Jung ME, et al. 2014. Where does HIT fit? An examination of the affective response to high- intensity intervals in comparison to continous moderate- and continuous vigorous-intensity exercise in the exercise intensity- affect continuum. PLoS ONE 9(12):e114541.

Bartlett JD, et al. 2011. High-intensity interval running is perceived to be more enjoyable than moderate-intensity continuous exercise: implications for exercise adherence. J Sports Sci 29:547-553.

Jung ME, et al. 2015. High-intensity interval training as an efficacious alternative to moderate-intensity continuous training for adults with prediabetes. J Diab Res 191595.

Knowles A, et al. 2015. Impact of low-volume, high-intensity interval training on maximal aerobic capacity, health-related quality of life and motivation to exercise in ageing men. AGE 37:25.

Martinez N, et al. 2015. Affective and enjoyment responses to high-intensity interval training in overweight-to-obese and insufficiently active adults. J Sport Exerc Psychol 37(2):138-49.

Goldfarb AH, et al. 1990. Plasma beta-endorphin concentration: response to intensity and duration of exercise. Med Sci Sports Exercs 22(2):241-4.

Kjaer M. 1989. Epinephrine and some other hormonal responses to exercise in man: with special reference to physical training. Int J Sports Med 10:2-15.

Lagenfeld ME, et al. 1987. Plasma beta-endorphin responses to one-hour bicycling and running at 60% vo2max. Med Sci Sports Exerc 19(2):83-6.

Draznin B, et al. 2012. Effect of Dietary Macronutrient Composition on AMPK and SIRT1 Expression and Activity in Human Skeletal Muscle. Horm Metab Res 44(09):650-655.

Cantó C, et al. 2010. Interdependence of AMPK and SIRT1 for metabolic adaptation to fasting and exercise in skeletal muscle. Cell Metab 11(3):213-219.

Vavvas D, et al. 1997. Contraction-induced changes in acetyl-CoA carboxylase and 5'-AMP-activated kinase in skeletal muscle. J Biol Chem. 272(20):13255-13261.

Winder WW, et al. 1996. Inactivation of acetyl-CoA carboxylase and activation of AMP-activated protein kinase in muscle during exercise. Am J Physiol. 270(2 Pt 1):E299-E304.

Rasmussen BB, et al. 1997. Effect of exercise intensity on skeletal muscle malonyl-CoA and acetyl-CoA carboxylase. J Appl Physiol. 1997;83(4):1104-1109.

Shackelford DB, et al. 2009. The LKB1-AMPK pathway: metabolism and growth control in tumour suppression. Nat Rev Cancer. 9(8):563-575.

Green AS, et al. 2010. The LKB1/AMPK signaling pathway has tumor suppressor activity in acute myeloid leukemia through the repression of mTOR-dependent oncogenic mRNA translation. Blood. 116(20):4262-4273.

Champ CE, et al. 2013. Nutrient Restriction and Radiation Therapy for Cancer Treatment: When Less Is More. Oncologist. 18(1):97-103.

Faubert B, et al. 2013. AMPK is a negative regulator of the Warburg effect and suppresses tumor growth in vivo. Cell Metab. 17(1):113-124.

Conclusion

Huffman KM, et al. 2014. Metabolite signatures of exercise training in human skeletal muscle relate to mitochondrial remodelling and cardiometabolic fitness. Diabetologia 57:2282-2295.

Costa P, et al. 2011. Acute Effects of Static Stretching on Peak Torque and the Hamstrings-to-Quadriceps Conventional and Functional Ratios. Scan J Med Sci Sport.

Esposito F, et al. 2011. Time Course of Stretching-Induced Changes in Mechanomyogram and Force Characteristics. J Electro Kin 21:795-802.

Esposito F, et al. 2012. Cycling Efficiency and Time to Exhaustion are Reduced After Acute Passive Stretching Administration. Scan J Med Sci Sport. 22:737-745.

Miyahara Y, et al. 2012. Effects of Proprioceptive Neuromuscular Facilitation Stretching and Static Stretching on Maximal Voluntary Contraction. J Strength Cond Res.

Pacheco L, et al. 2011. The Acute Effects of Different Stretching Exercises on Jump Performance. J Strength Cond Res.

Crow J, et al. 2012. Low Load Exercises Targeting the Gluteal Muscle Group acutely Enhance Explosive Power Output in Elite Athletes. J Strength Cond Res.

Schmidtbleicher D, et al. 2012. Effects of Functional Exercises in the Warm-up On Sprint Performance. J Strength Cond Res.

Safran M, et al. 1989. Warm-up and muscular injury prevention. Sport Med 4:239-49.

Martin B, et al. 1975. Effect of warm-up on metabolic responses to strenuous exercise. Med Sci Sport Exerc 7:146-49.

Hart, L. 2005. Effect of stretching on sport injury risk: A review. Clin J Sports Med 15:371-78.

44353926R00183

Made in the USA
Middletown, DE
04 June 2017